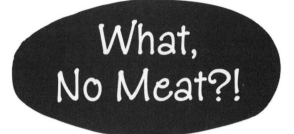

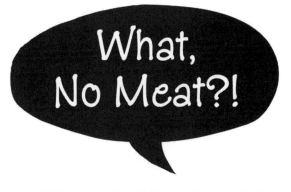

What to do When Your Kid Becomes a Vegetarian

**Debra Halperin Poneman
and
Emily Anderson Greene**

ECWPRESS
ecwpress.com

Published by ECW PRESS
2120 Queen Street East, Suite 200, Toronto, Ontario, Canada M4E 1E2

NATIONAL LIBRARY OF CANADA CATALOGUING IN PUBLICATION DATA

Poneman, Debra Halperin
What, No Meat?!: what to do when your kid becomes a vegetarian/
Debra Halperin Poneman and Emily Anderson Greene.

Includes index.
ISBN 1-55022-579-0
1. Vegetarian children. 2. Vegetarianism. 3. Vegetarian cookery.
I. Anderson Greene, Emily II. Title.

TX392.P65 2003   613.2'62'083   C2003-902206-4

Acquisition & production: Emma McKay, Copy editor: Dallas Harrison
Text design & typesetting: Guylaine Régimbald — Solo Design
Cover design: Paul Hodgson, Illustrations: Brian Gable
Printing: Transcontinental

Diligent efforts have been made to contact copyright holders; please
excuse any inadvertent errors or omissions, but if anyone has been
unintentionally omitted, the publisher would be pleased to receive
notification and make acknowledgements in future printings.

This book is set in DTL Nobel

The publication of *What, No Meat?!* has been generously supported
by the Canada Council, by the Government of Ontario through the
Ontario Media Development Corporation's Ontario Book Initiative,
by the Ontario Arts Council, and by the Government of Canada through
the Book Publishing Industry Development Program. Canadä

DISTRIBUTION

CANADA: Jaguar Book Group, 100 Armstrong Avenue,
Georgetown, Ontario L7G 5S4

UNITED STATES: Independent Publishers Group, 814 North Franklin Street,
Chicago, Illinois 60610

EUROPE: Turnaround Publisher Services, Unit 3, Olympia Trading Estate,
Coburg Road, Wood Green, London N2Z 6T2

AUSTRALIA AND NEW ZEALAND: Wakefield Press, 1 The Parade West
(Box 2266), Kent Town, South Australia 5071

PRINTED AND BOUND IN CANADA

ECW PRESS
ecwpress.com

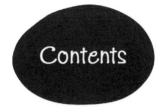

Contents

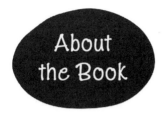

About the Book

This book is dedicated to our mothers,
whose main ingredient was always love.

It's a new millennium, and teenage vegetarianism has become an accepted lifestyle as well as a growing economic force throughout the world. In fact, despite the dot com bomb, the stock of Whole Foods Markets International has hardly fluctuated in the past seven years. According to the US Census Bureau, there are over one million school-age children who never eat meat, fish, or fowl and millions more who significantly limit their meat consumption.

But as commonplace as vegetarian kids and teens are, some things have not changed — most notably the resistance with which their parents almost universally react. And I don't blame them. Parents are concerned about the health of their children, and the advertising media, especially for the powerful beef and dairy industries, have done a formidable job of convincing us that meat and milk are essential for good health and sound nutrition. How many magazines do you open and see a picture of a top celebrity, glowing with health and smiling out at you, with the caption "Got spinach?"

As concerned as parents are about their children's health, they are perhaps more concerned that this new "vegetarian thing" will be a major intrusion on their own lifestyles. Parents today are already overwrought trying to balance kids, careers, bills, exercise, aging parents, and who knows what else. No wonder they feel that having to learn to cook and shop in a whole new "vegetarian way" just might tip the scales.

What, No Meat?! is written for the harried house parent willing to make the effort to accommodate a child's decision to become a vegetarian but who wants the whole thing to be as quick and simple as possible. This book doesn't overwhelm readers with information about how the Zulus in Africa drank beet juice and lived to be 200. Instead, it offers simple, sound facts that will allay parental fears about nutritional deficiencies in a child's vegetarian diet. The book doesn't include recipes that start with shelling your own peas or kerneling your own corn; it simply suggests that you throw a soy dog on the barbecue next to the Oscar Meyer's and call it a day. And, especially for those of you who love to cook, an adventurous recipe section offers vegetarian recipes your whole family will love.

When parents of new vegetarians go to the bookstore to figure out where to begin, they will quickly notice that there are more vegetarian cookbooks than they could sift through in a year. But a cookbook is not what parents need—they need a *handbook* like this one because it's not just the recipes that are important.

Parents need to know how to effortlessly accommodate their vegetarian child while still providing for the needs of the other members of the family. They need to know they can still go out for dinner—and where. They need to know the proper etiquette for when the boss invites the whole family over for his wife's famous stuffed Cornish hens. They need to know what to do on Thanksgiving. And they need to know how to support their child's transition to a vegetarian diet in a way that is easy, peaceful, and hopefully even fun.

What, No Meat?! is easy to read. Important points are illustrated with easy-to-decipher charts and graphs. Because there are different types of vegetarianism, icons lead readers directly to the information pertinent to their child. Additionally, eye-catching illustrations at the beginning of each chapter offer humorous insights into parents' concerns.

What, No Meat?! isn't a treatise. Statistical overload isn't the aim. Sure, the book includes recipes as well as compelling evidence of the healthfulness of a vegetarian diet, but only what parents truly need to know—and from sources they already trust, such as the American Dietetic Association, American Heart Association, and American Council on Nutrition.

Finally, although this book is written in Debra's voice, it was 100% a collaborative effort—and, if truth be known, Emily is the goddess of the kitchen and the one responsible for researching, creating, and testing all the delicious recipes. With each author contributing her expertise, you'll benefit not only from Debra's experience as the mother of two vegetarian children and the vegetarian daughter of parents who did their best to accommodate her lifestyle over 30 years ago, but also from Emily's more recent conversion to a vegetarian lifestyle—not to mention her vegetarian pregnancy!

When we told our own mothers about this book, they both said they wished we had written it years ago but could definitely still use it today. We're sure that no such book exists, because if it did we would have bought it for our moms a long time ago.

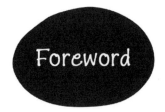

Foreword

In 1985, when I coauthored *Fit for Life*, my goal was to assist readers in understanding the choices they could make that would lead to healthier living. I am still committed to that goal and continue to bring the message of good health to people throughout the world. One of the ways I do this is by supporting friends and colleagues who are working to make a difference.

When my good friends Debra and Emily asked me to write the foreword to *What, No Meat?!* I felt honored to support their efforts. Educating people about vegetarianism is extremely important to me. Even more important is educating parents of vegetarian children since the children are the future of our world. Having raised a vegetarian child in the era before this was a popular choice, I fully understand the challenges both children and their parents face.

This informative and practical guidebook for conscious and concerned parents is so important and timely. It is written not only with the children's best interests in mind but also with those of the whole family. It offers compassion, encouragement, and indispensable wisdom of the highest spiritual nature to those who are bringing up the next generation . . . and shaping the future of our world.

The thought of raising a vegetarian child may seem overwhelming, but let me remind you that you are not alone. Today there are over 2.5 million parents of strict vegetarian kids in the United States and many million more whose children are semi-vegetarian. With rising concerns over growth hormones, genetic engineering, and food-borne illnesses, the food industry is projecting increases of one million or more vegetarians a year. This trend is evidenced by the growth in popularity of natural food stores, vegetarian choices in restaurants from the most elegant to the most convenient, the proliferation of vegetarian magazines and cookbooks, and the abundance of vegetarian products in mainstream grocery stores (and even coupons for products such as Boca Burgers in the Sunday paper!)

I would like to congratulate you on reading this book, and I must add that you are in the best of hands. The truth is that many parents are taken by surprise and are not sure whether or not to support their child's vegetarian decision. This book will help you to weather the whole process, from the initial shock through the stages of listening, understanding, and then hopefully accepting and supporting the child's decision.

On a practical level, this book is your godsend. With a combination of useful information and simple yet delicious recipes, it is the perfect starter kit. With the latest in dietary and nutritional research, you will be armed with the facts about what really constitutes a healthy vegetarian diet. This book also addresses a busy parent's approach to menu planning, shopping, and cooking, with simple tips for a vegetarian kitchen and explanations that will take the mystery out of tofu and tempeh. Debra and Emily have marked the recipes with icons to identify eggs and dairy, so that parents of both vegetarians and strict vegans will find them useful. I also appreciate that information is included on the more delicate issues of living a vegetarian life, such as proper etiquette and how your child's decision impacts the future of our planet. All the while, the book is easy to read and free of heavy dogma and data. *What, No Meat?!* contains just the information you need to know as a dedicated and caring parent.

On a personal level, I second Debra and Emily's entreaty that you be as supportive as possible. From one parent to another, I know that it's not easy to accept such a drastic change, especially since we are still predominantly a carnivorous society. But the research is compelling, even irrefutable, that a well-balanced vegetarian diet will lead to lifelong improved health and well-being.

If I were parenting younger children today, I would be very cautious about the food I put on their plates. From fast food to school lunches, children are eating foods that do not nourish their bodies — or their souls. It is up to you as a parent to give them the most nourishing food you can at home, and this book will help you to do just that. Good health is both their birthright and yours. Anything you can do to help your children enjoy good health will pay dividends far into the future. This book is a great place to start.

About Marilyn Diamond

For over two decades, Marilyn Diamond has been a pioneer in leading people to higher health awareness. She is the co-author of the *New York Times* best-seller *Fit for Life*, *Fit for Life 2*, and *Fitonics* and the author of *A New Way of Eating*, *The American Vegetarian Cookbook*, and *Recipes for Life*. She is president of Enlightenment 101 and cofounder of the Power of Love Foundation. Her organizations offer cutting-edge body-mind-spirit educational materials and seminars to clients around the world. Her focus remains on empowering others to take responsibility for their health and happiness. Her new books, *Marilyn Diamond's Fast and Easy Weight Loss Solution* and *Spiritually Fit for Life*, culminate 30 years of research, lecturing, and counseling in the philosophy she herself lives and coaches others to live every day.

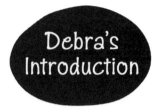

Debra's
Introduction

Your daughter comes home with triple-pierced ears, and you're relieved that at least it isn't her tongue. Your son shaves his head, but as shocked as you are you're glad he didn't dye his hair purple. You think you've handled it all, and now this, the *v* word. Your child has decided to become a vegetarian.

No more Ballpark Franks? No more pepperoni pizza? Not even KFC! How are you going to explain this one to Grandma?

More than 30 years ago, when I announced to my family that I was no longer going to eat meat, they looked at me like I had two heads. In 1970, I was considered quite an anomaly in the affluent northern suburbs of Chicago. Not only was my mom sure I was now going to die of malnutrition, but, when our family was invited out and she was forced to tell someone in her circle that her seemingly normal daughter was a vegetarian, you'd have thought she was telling them that I had leprosy or was pregnant—with twins.

Fast-forward to 2003, and vegetarianism has become a major trend among North American youth, and now it has infiltrated your kitchen. Don't panic, Mom and Dad, it could be worse. Unlike serpentine tattoos and Hollywood-induced teen anorexia, this trend is one you can live with, and this book will show you how.

I know that vegetarianism may defy your primal survival instincts. After all, there's been meat next to the potatoes on your son's plate since he went off the Gerber's—and look how healthy he is. But with meat-borne diseases reaching epidemic proportions, the large amounts of antibiotics and salmonella being found in our poultry, PCBs turning up in our fish, and medical professionals warning us that our teenagers' arteries look like those of 50 or 60 year olds, you should probably be celebrating rather than trying to figure out where you went wrong.

This is most likely not the first time your child has adopted a position you don't understand, and I'm sure it won't be the last. The difference is that this decision includes you big-time because you're the cook. You're the one who does the shopping. You're the master of the barbecue grill. And you don't have a clue about the difference between tempeh and tofu and probably don't really care. And aren't all vegetarians weird anyway?

So what's a parent to do?

In this book, you'll learn how a balanced vegetarian diet is healthful, even for kids, and how cooking for your vegetarian child isn't the hassle you imagine. Not only will you gain the tools to make your family's transition a smooth and happy one, but you will also learn some facts about our food supply, the direction of agriculture, and compelling medical evidence that just may inspire you to try a vegetarian diet yourself.

Your child's decision to become a vegetarian has the potential to be a source of disharmony and division in your family, or it can be the beginning of a fun and exciting family adventure. I don't have to tell you that, if you resist or, worse yet, belittle your child's decision, nothing positive will come from it. So be supportive, and give vegetarianism a chance. And one more thing: don't worry if they're getting enough protein!

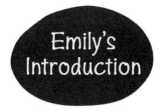

Emily's
Introduction

When Debra asked me to help her write this book, I was honored. I never expected to cowrite a book with such an established expert on health and nutrition. And, quite frankly, I was delighted to see how our relationship had progressed since we first met when I was—*are you ready for this?*—her children's babysitter!

It's true! We met when I was a freshman in college, and from the moment I set foot in the Poneman household I noticed that they did things—well, how can I say?—a little differently. Seeing the organic soy milk in their refrigerator and the vegan peanut butter cups in their cupboard, I knew Debra was no ordinary mother. She had a passion for holistic health and well-being that I found inspiring.

I quickly learned that Debra was a walking university. Within months, she had educated me about organic produce, toxic household chemicals, and natural body care products. I was amazed to discover that her two healthy children had never taken an antibiotic in their lives. I was most excited to learn that she had been a vegetarian since the age of 18.

Many times over the next several years, as more of her friends' children and her children's friends became vegetarians, Debra mentioned her desire to write this book. Over and over again, she bemoaned the fact that she had no time to do it. Then one day she had the brilliant idea to ask me to write it with her!

Together we bring a unique multigenerational perspective to the topic of teen vegetarianism. In fact, we represent two different sides of the vegetarian spectrum. While Debra became a vegetarian in the politically charged 1970s and now lives in the world of soccer party barbecues, I became a vegetarian in the health-obsessed 1990s and now live in the world of new parents and young professionals. Our different experiences and motivations for vegetarian living allow us to address a broader range of issues you will encounter with your child.

This is important because no two people have the same vegetarian experience. For example, unlike Debra, I never had a defining moment in which I "became" a vegetarian. Although I was raised in a family that ate meat, I never really liked it. In high school, after my grandfather died of a heart attack, I began to read every book I could find on health and nutrition. It didn't take long to discover that meat of all kinds is linked to heart disease, obesity, and even cancer. After much research, I decided that a well-balanced vegetarian diet is the optimal fuel for the human body.

When I began to leave meat off the plate, my parents were very supportive. They knew my choice was motivated by a desire to stay in excellent health. In fact, through my high school years, I remember having several interesting discussions with my family about the health benefits of a vegetarian lifestyle. As I explained to them, for me becoming vegetarian was pure logic. Vegetables do not have cholesterol or high levels of saturated fat. It was a no-brainer.

I never thought my beliefs were controversial. In fact, I had a hard time seeing why being a vegetarian was such a big deal to so many people. From firsthand experience, I learned that, if someone offered me a hamburger and I didn't eat it because I didn't like meat, that seemed to be okay. But if I didn't eat it because I was a *vegetarian*, my choice suddenly became contentious.

It took years for me to understand that most people presume being vegetarian carries *political* connotations. This isn't always true. It wasn't until college that I began to meet people who led politically motivated "vegetarian lifestyles," and I found these people to be a bit extreme at first. Suddenly I came in contact with individuals who not only made vegetarian food choices but also refused to wear leather of any kind, wouldn't use laundry detergent that had been tested on animals, and wouldn't even eat frozen yogurt! I began to see how wide the vegetarian spectrum stretches and where I fell on that line.

I am a complete vegetarian. I do not eat meat of any kind, and I rarely eat dairy products. Despite all the knowledge I've gained about the superior health benefits of a vegetarian diet, I try not to preach my preferences to every passerby. Instead, I like to talk about the factual health benefits of a vegetarian diet. And I hope that my own good health will be motivation for others to consider cutting back on meat.

I try not to make my food preferences an obsession. I recently got married to a wonderful man who is not a vegetarian. Although he rarely eats red meat, he does occasionally enjoy chicken and fish. Even though we don't cook meat in our home, I have no objection to my spouse ordering meat when we go out for dinner. And, truthfully, if he wanted to throw some hot wings on the grill, I certainly wouldn't let a piece of chicken harm our relationship. Both my husband and I believe that, as important as it is, eating is not all of life. That being said, I do enjoy showing him that vegetarian meals can be both visually appealing and tasty. I love finding new recipes to keep his taste buds excited, and he is starting to prefer the vegetarian meals we eat at home to any food—chicken, fish, or otherwise—we eat outside the house.

My husband also appreciates the improved health and vitality he now experiences as a result of his near-vegetarian diet. And as we start a family of our own, we'll keep well-being at the forefront. We've discussed whether or not to raise our children as vegetarians, and we agree that we will limit their consumption of meat. And, yes, I even had a vegetarian pregnancy.

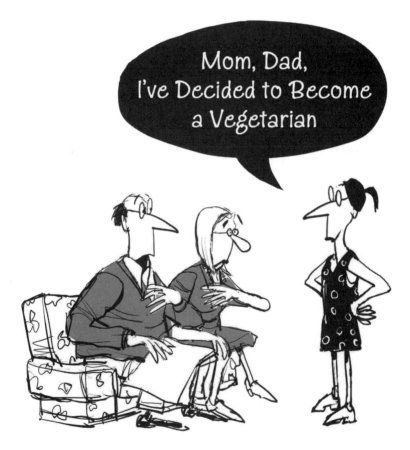

CHAPTER 1

Starting off on the Right Foot

I remember clearly the day I came home and announced to my parents that I had, after careful thought, decided to become a vegetarian. My mom glanced at me skeptically and, without skipping a beat, said, "That's nice, but Daddy has some skirt steaks on the grill, so why don't you wait until tomorrow?" That sounded like a good idea to me.

But as delicious as those steaks were, I was determined to become a vegetarian. It was 1970, the era of peace and love, and killing in any form was out of the question. Those barbecued skirt steaks became, in essence, my last supper.

Times have definitely changed. Although many young people today are still becoming vegetarians for humanitarian reasons, others are doing so for different reasons. It may be that they care deeply about the future of our planet and believe that, by eating lower on the food chain, they can contribute to that future. Perhaps they have familiarized themselves with the health benefits of a vegetarian diet. They may have been moved by a TV exposé on the horrible conditions animals are subjected to from the time of birth so that they can be displayed on our supermarket shelves. Maybe they went without eating meat for a few weeks at summer camp and discovered they felt a whole lot better. Or perhaps they have no concrete reason at all, other than an inner voice telling them it's what they want, and they're choosing to follow that inner voice. That's what you've always taught them to do, isn't it?

If you don't know why your children, growing up in your home, made this decision, my suggestion is to ask them. Take a moment to sit down and discuss their reasons, and listen to what they say with full attention. Hear them out before you tell them all the reasons you think becoming a vegetarian is a bad idea. You just might be surprised at how rational and mature their thinking is. Understanding your children's motivation will help you give them what they need most—your support.

How to Be Supportive

The last thing your child needs is to be put down, belittled, or forced to justify her decision. Trust me, since we still live in a predominantly meat-eating society, your child is going to have to justify her food choices again and again—probably for the rest of her life. From you, she'd just like some acceptance and respect.

Think back on your own life and those moments when your worldview was about to collide with your parents' long-held beliefs. It may have been when you told them you were changing your major—from premed to acting. What about when you decided not to go into the family business? Or the day you told them you were getting married—to someone of a different religion. At those moments, all you wanted was for your parents to react with understanding. You didn't necessarily expect them to agree, but you hoped they would see that you were following your heart—and maybe even be proud of you for it.

By becoming a vegetarian, your child is doing what she believes is right. Who knows if this decision will last for a day, a year, or the rest of her life? But it doesn't matter. Right now it's important to her, and she wants your support, just as you did from your parents.

And it's important to restrain yourself when tempted to do what I've seen many parents do—relish the moment when your child breaks her conviction. "I told you so" is not what she needs to hear.

I'll never forget the afternoon at an outdoor party in Cambridge, Massachusetts. My brother was graduating from Harvard, and while scrutinizing the hors d'oeuvres tray I connected with another "little sister" who, I discovered, was also a vegetarian. We were surrounded by family and friends, and the food was flowing by at a furious pace.

We soon became engaged in an intense political conversation, and she absentmindedly toothpicked and downed a tiny Swedish meatball. Well, you would have thought the Harvard Rowing Team had just won the Ivy League championship by the victory celebration that ensued. I was amazed to see that her family and friends, who seemed so pleasant, were secretly so eager to see her falter in her commitment.

Save it, please. It's rude and inappropriate. No one would tease or taunt someone who goes off her weight-loss diet. No one would rejoice when someone breaks a commitment not to smoke a cigarette or drink an alcoholic beverage. Don't make this into a power struggle. Much more important than what your child chooses to eat is that it's eaten in an atmosphere of love and harmony.

And if you're going to make the effort to support her lifestyle, she should respect yours. Becoming a vegetarian does not give your child the license to forget her manners or act like she is "holier than thou." If she does any of that "meat is so gross" stuff at your dinner table, you have full permission to ground her.

It's Really Not Uncommon

Perhaps you feel that, by choosing to become a vegetarian, your child is separating himself from the mainstream of society and joining a small group of renegades reminiscent of the long-haired commune dwellers of the 1960s. You're concerned that this choice will make his life difficult because so much of daily activity is centered on eating. Nothing could be further from the truth. These days non-meat eaters versus meat eaters are as common as decaf versus regular coffee drinkers.

As our population becomes increasingly heart and health conscious, the number of people becoming vegetarians is growing at an astounding rate. According to a Vegetarian Resource Group (VRG) Zogby poll (see www.vrg.org), more than half the US population has either eliminated or dramatically reduced the intake of red meat in their diets.

Don't tell me that during the mad cow scare you didn't hesitate when you picked up that package of ground beef. Perhaps you thought twice and chose ground turkey instead. And the last time the office ordered in pizza, did you not stare apprehensively at that sausage before picking it from the cheese?

Vegetarianism is not a new concept. It has been practiced by many notable individuals throughout history, including Albert Einstein, Henry Ford, George Bernard Shaw, Leo Tolstoy, and Michelangelo. In more recent times, Doris Day, Mary Tyler Moore, Yehudi Menuhin, all four Beatles, Coretta Scott King, Jerry Seinfeld, Steve Martin, Phylicia Rashad, Ashley Judd, Carl Lewis, Chelsea Clinton, and Bob Barker have been vegetarians. Want a few more? Include Saint Francis of Assisi, Dr. Benjamin Spock, and Mr. Rogers. Nobel prize winners, Olympic gold medalists, and saints. Not bad company!

Almost three years after going vegan, Alicia Silverstone says she couldn't be happier. "I can't tell you how much better I feel," she says. "I did it solely for moral reasons but can feel the results in every aspect of my life. I sleep better, my skin has never been so clear, and I never have to worry about weight again."

It's Really Not That Difficult

Okay, so you don't really care about famous vegetarians, but you do care about how your child's decision is going to affect you. One of your concerns is that it is going to be a major time-consuming intrusion on you and the rest of the family. Juggling shopping and cooking with all your other responsibilities is hard enough, and now this! But as you'll see in chapter 3, you can make this transition with less effort than it took you to switch from your old electric typewriter to your new PC. Once you get the hang of it, preparing food for your vegetarian child will be second nature. I'm not saying it won't take any extra effort or thought, but shouldn't feeding any child require time and thought?

And one more thing: you know how you've been lamenting lately that time has flown by so quickly, and you wish you'd made more of those days when your children actually wanted your attention—when their idea of a good time was to spend the day with you? Well, guess what, lucky you, they want your attention and need you again. This could be a great opportunity to share something with your children before they drift away into their own lives forever. You can shop with them, plan menus with them, cook with them, and just have fun together. I know a lot of parents who would love to be in your shoes.

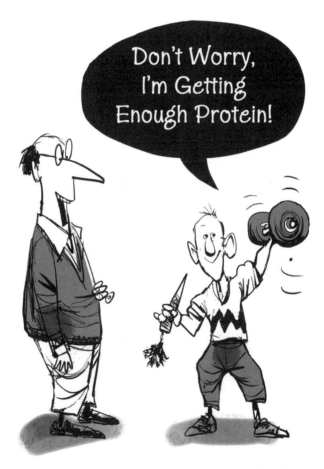

CHAPTER 2

Nutritional Myths and Realities

As parents, from the moment you see that second pink line appear on the in-home pregnancy test, you want only two things for your children: for them to be healthy and happy.

You get the best prenatal care and make sure your vitamins have the necessary amounts of folic acid and iron. You wouldn't dream of touching a cigarette or a glass of wine. *What to Expect When You're Expecting* never leaves your bedside table. And when that child enters the world and you gently hold that baby in your arms, there is nothing more important to you than the well-being of this tiny angel now in your care.

You have your children's best interests in mind when you decide between breast milk and formula. You carefully determine when they're ready for their first solid food. You give them their little TV character vitamins, keep the sweets to a minimum, and only give in to the drive-thru window when you're really in a pinch. You may even hang a picture of the food pyramid on your refrigerator and try to make sure that, at least for dinner, they have one food from each important category.

Now they've made it through adolescence, and you're proud of the job you've done. They've turned out at least relatively healthy and happy. But if the truth be known, you sometimes forgot to give them their little vitamins, and the food pyramid got covered up by the soccer pictures a long time ago. But it's really not your fault; you're just soooo busy, and they're never home anyway, and even President Reagan said ketchup is a vegetable, *and what's so wrong with McDonald's?*

Welcome to the real world. You're not a bad parent; you're just a typical parent of the 21st century trying to do what's best for your children.

In an ideal world, our children would crave seven servings of vegetables and five servings of fruit each day, but we know that with our fast-food pace of life we have little control over what they eat most of the time. We just have to accept it, cross our fingers, and marvel over how healthy they are on only one serving of vegetables — and that's the green pepper on their pizza.

So why is it that, when your child tells you she's decided to become a vegetarian, some frantic survival instinct kicks in, and you're positive she's going to die of malnutrition? Why is it that you are suddenly obsessed with proper nutrition, more so now than when macaroni and cheese was her primary sustenance? The phrase "protein deficiency" now haunts you, and images of malnourished, paper-thin children keep you awake at night. You're not alone; this near panic is a universal reaction.

I've been a vegetarian for over 30 years, and not only am I one of the healthiest people around, but also, when I tell people my age, their jaws drop. Yet my mom is still absolutely positive that I'm not getting enough protein.

Some Surprising Facts about Nutritional Myths

Old ideas die hard, and advertising dollars rule the world. Many North Americans still cling to nutritional myths that belie the benefits of vegetarian eating. They don't know that, in many cases, these myths are based on out-of-date information, misunderstanding of scientific concepts, or research funded by industries that benefit from our belief in these myths. And even when people accept that plant-based diets are okay for adults, there is still a predominant reluctance in our society to accept them for kids and teens.

If you're like most parents of new vegetarians, your main question is "Can my child's growing body get the nutrients and calories it needs without meat?" According to experts from the American Dietetic Association (ADA), the answer is, with simple planning, yes. "Vegetarian diets can be healthful for people of all ages," says Julie Covington, a Gastonia, North Carolina, registered dietitian and chair of ADA's vegetarian nutrition practice group. "Research shows a carefully planned vegetarian diet can be nutritionally adequate and healthful for children from infants to teenagers."

It's really not difficult to provide a child with a healthy, well-balanced vegetarian diet—and that includes getting enough protein!

The Protein Myth

There's hardly another nutritional myth so insidious yet so enduring as that which encourages us to believe that consuming mass quantities of protein is essential for good health, strong bones, and normal growth. Rooted in antiquity, and fueled by studies funded by the National Beef Association, among others, this myth frightens us into accepting as fact that we need to consume a huge amount of protein. Moreover, it scares us into thinking that we'd better get it one of two ways: either by eating the flesh of dead animals or by consuming their milk. Without beef and dairy, we will certainly become lethargic, scrawny, and weak, or so we are taught.

But wait, it has to be true! My fourth-grade teacher told me so! Never mind that some of the teaching materials she utilized were probably supplied to her free of charge by the National Dairy Council, the foremost supplier of "nutritional education" materials to classrooms in the United States.

No parent in his or her right mind would dispute that adequate protein is vital to a child's health. Protein makes up 50 percent of the non-water components of our bodies, including skin, hair, nails, tendons, muscles, and even the organic framework of our bones. Some proteins are necessary to regulate hormones, and even hemoglobin is built from protein. Perhaps most importantly, protein synthesis is needed to form antibodies to fight bacterial and viral infections.

It is not the necessity of protein that is in question; it is the quantity and source of that protein. The amount of protein we actually need to ensure that all our bodily systems function optimally is only about 56 grams per day for the average man,

44 grams per day for the average woman, and similar amounts for children and teens.

Recommended Dietary Allowances (RDAs) for Protein

Ages	Female	Male
11 to 14 years old	46 g	45 g
15 to 18 years old	44 g	59 g
19 to 24 years old	46 g	53 g

Excess protein—in particular animal protein—actually places strain on many of the body's systems and is linked to accelerated aging. Scientists have discovered that the body uses protein less efficiently when we take in more protein than required and more efficiently when we eat at or near our ideal requirement.

Do you know that most North Americans already consume *twice* their recommended daily allowance of protein? Do you know that science has linked high-protein diets to obesity, liver disease, and kidney failure? Do you know that our bodies have no means of storing excess protein? The more excess protein in the diet, the greater the incidence of negative calcium balance —hence the greater the loss of calcium from bones, resulting in osteoporosis. With all the evidence to the contrary, it's amazing how many people still believe they'll feel a lot better if they just wash down a juicy steak with a tall glass of milk.

Meat protein is not the only viable source for meeting our daily protein requirement. Nor is it the healthiest source. It's not that animal protein cannot be utilized by the body or that it doesn't build muscle mass. It does. But it does not accomplish the job any more effectively than plant protein.

The belief that meat protein is superior to plant protein is undermined by medical science. The data deflates the hype. Take a look at the charts below, and one thing will be evident: plant-based proteins can offer the same quantity of protein as animal-derived proteins (and with fewer calories, less fat, and no cholesterol).

Plant-Based Protein Sources

Food	Amount	Protein	Cholesterol
Tempeh	1 cup	31 g	0 mg
Seitan	4 oz	19–31 g	0 mg
Soybeans, cooked	1 cup	29 g	0 mg
Veggie dog	1 link	13–26 g	0 mg
Veggie burger	1 patty	8–24 g	0 mg
Lentils, cooked	1 cup	18 g	0 mg
Tofu, firm	4 oz	9–15 g	0 mg
Kidney beans, cooked	1 cup	15 g	0 mg
Black beans, cooked	1 cup	15 g	0 mg
Bagel	1 medium	9 g	0 mg
Peas, cooked	1 cup	9 g	0 mg
Peanut butter	2 tbsp	8 g	0 mg
Spaghetti, cooked	1 cup	7 g	0 mg
Spinach, cooked	1 cup	6 g	0 mg
Broccoli, cooked	1 cup	5 g	0 mg
Whole-wheat bread	2 slices	5 g	0 mg
Cashews	1/4 cup	5 g	0 mg
Brown rice, cooked	1 cup	5 g	0 mg
Potato	1 medium	4 g	0 mg

Source: USDA Nutrient Database for Standard Reference

Animal-Based Protein Sources

Food	Amount	Protein	Cholesterol
Chicken, baked	3 oz	28 g	95 mg
Pork roast	3 oz	25 g	79 mg
Sirloin steak	3 oz	24 g	84 mg
Flounder, baked	3 oz	21 g	53 mg
Ground beef, lean	3 oz	20 g	89 mg
Cow's milk	1 cup	8 g	20 mg
Cheddar cheese	1 oz	7 g	30 mg
Egg	1 large	6 g	212.5 mg

Source: USDA Nutrient Database for Standard Reference

Because of lower fat and cholesterol content, plant protein is not linked to heart disease, liver disease, kidney failure, cancer, or other known killers, but it does add the extra benefit of fiber, antioxidants, and high vitamin and mineral content. No wonder each successive year more people are becoming vegetarians. In fact, the food industry is projecting increases of one million new vegetarians a year for the next several years in the United States alone.

Still worried? Take a look at how simple it is to obtain an adequate amount of protein from solely a plant-based diet.

What if My Child Eats . . .

FOOD	CALORIES	PROTEIN
BREAKFAST		
1 cup orange juice	109	1.7 g
1 cup cooked oatmeal	144	5.4 g
1 oz sunflower seeds	80	3.5 g
1 tbsp brown sugar	52	0 g
3 tbsp raisins	87	.9 g
LUNCH		
2 tbsp peanut butter	172	7.8 g
2 slices whole-wheat bread	112	4.8 g
1 tbsp jelly	38	.01 g
1 apple	87	.03 g
2 carrots, small	42	1.1 g
DINNER		
1 tofu dog	95	15.6 g
1 enriched bun	110	3 g
1 small ear of corn	77	3 g
1 cup peas	58	4 g
1 cup apple juice	245	0 g
SNACK		
1 banana	108	1 g
1 box animal crackers	254	4 g
1 soy milk drink box	120	4 g
Total	**1,990**	**59.8 g**
RDA Requirements	**2,000**	**44.0 g**

Almost all foods offer some protein, except for fruits, fats, and alcohol. As long as your child doesn't subsist solely on bananas, butter, and beer, your concerns about protein should be allayed.

The Calcium Myth

Another common myth is that vegetarian children's bones and teeth will not be as strong as those of their nonvegetarian counterparts because of a lack of calcium.

There is no disputing the importance of calcium in your child's diet, since bone density is determined in adolescence and young adulthood. Thus, it is important to include three or more good sources of calcium in a growing child's diet so that a minimum of 1,000 to 1,200 milligrams are consumed each day. How is it possible for child vegetarians, particularly vegans, who avoid dairy and eggs, to consume enough calcium to prevent this deficiency? Shouldn't they drink milk at least?

Maybe not. Dairy products are certainly abundant in calcium, and three servings of dairy will usually get you to the 1,000 milligram mark. But with dairy you also have the potential for a high intake of saturated fats that could lead not only to weight gain but also to heart disease, hypertension, and, some suggest, even cancer. You might also develop dairy-related allergies and digestive problems.

Dairy Sources of Calcium

Item	Serving	Calories	Fat	Protein	Calcium
Plain yogurt	8 oz	143.5	3.5 g	12 g	414 mg
Skim milk with vitamin A	1 cup	85.5	0.5 g	8.5 g	302 mg
2% milk with vitamin A	1 cup	121	4.5 g	8 g	296 mg
Whole milk	1 cup	150	8 g	8 g	291 mg
Sour cream	1 cup	400	48 g	7.5 g	267 mg
Cheddar cheese	1 oz	114	9.5 g	7 g	204 mg
American cheese	1 oz	106.5	9 g	6.5 g	174 mg
2% cottage cheese	1 cup	202.5	4.5 g	31 g	155 mg
Mozzarella cheese	1 oz	80	6 g	5.5 g	146 mg
Frozen yogurt	1/2 cup	115	4.5 g	3 g	106 mg
Ice cream	1/2 cup	142.5	7.5 g	2.5 g	72 mg
Butter	1 tbsp	102	11.5 g	0 g	3 mg

Source: USDA — Nutrient Data Lab (Sept. 1996).
All data rounded to nearest 0.5.

Meat itself contains no calcium. And, as already mentioned, a diet high in animal protein can actually contribute to calcium excretion, thus promoting osteoporosis and bone loss. The average measurable bone loss of female meat eaters at age 65 is 35 percent compared with 18 percent for female vegetarians.

Vegetarian diets offer many excellent sources of calcium. Tofu processed with calcium sulfate, green leafy vegetables such as spinach and broccoli, and dried fruits and beans all contain high levels of calcium. Also, you can purchase enriched foods such as calcium-fortified orange juice, cereals such as Total, and breads as a way to boost calcium intake.

Nondairy Sources of Calcium

Item	Serving	Calories	Fat	Protein	Calcium
Calcium-fortified OJ	8 oz	110	0	2 g	300 mg
Soft tofu	4 oz	93	4.6 g	9.3 g	300mg
Calcium-fortified soy milk	8 oz	120	2 g	4 g	250 mg
Broccoli	1 cup	85	1 g	9 g	178 mg
Kidney beans	1 cup	220	0 g	16 g	144 mg
Figs	5 med	320	0 g	8 g	135 mg
Tempeh	1 cup	100–120	0 g	10–12 g	77 mg
Plain bagel	1 half	150	1 g	2 g	27 mg
Regular white pita	1 small	77	0.5 g	2.5 g	24 mg
Brown rice, cooked	1 cup	218.5	1.5 g	4.5 g	20 mg
Enriched white bread	1 slice	54	0.5 g	2 g	16 mg
Enriched wheat bread	1 slice	65	1 g	2 g	11 mg
Fresh spinach	2 oz	74	0.5 g	3 g	11 mg
Spaghetti, cooked	2 oz	74.5	0.5 g	3 g	4 mg

If you are a parent who believes in supplementation, another foolproof way to ensure adequate calcium intake is to add a calcium supplement to your child's daily regime. There are many delicious, chewable calcium supplements on the market that provide 50 percent or more of a young person's calcium requirement.

Finally, as vital as calcium is for growing children, the National Academy of Sciences actually warns that there are "tolerable upper intake levels" (ULs) for calcium. These are the maximum daily levels unlikely to pose risks of adverse effects such as kidney stones and impaired absorption of iron, zinc, and magnesium. The UL for calcium is 2,500 milligrams.

The Iron Myth

Iron is the most abundant mineral found in blood. The most important function of iron is in the production of hemoglobin, the part of the blood that carries oxygen throughout your body. Iron is also essential for proper growth, for maintaining a healthy immune system, and for energy production.

The iron requirements of teenagers are relatively high — and higher for girls than boys because they lose iron each month when they menstruate. The suggested minimum daily requirement of iron for girls ages 11 to 24 is 15 milligrams; for boys in the same age range, it is 12 milligrams. Yet the average American diet, vegetarian and nonvegetarian alike, contains only 6 milligrams of iron.

Iron-deficiency anemia is the most common childhood nutritional problem affecting one in six children and 10 to 25 percent of the general US population, mostly females. According to the US National Library of Medicine, the causes of iron deficiency are varied and include too little iron in the diet, poor absorption of iron by the body, and loss of blood (often from heavy menstrual bleeding). Iron-deficiency anemia develops slowly after the normal stores of iron have been depleted in the body and in bone marrow.

A common assumption is that iron deficiency is the direct result of a lack of red meat. You may be surprised to learn that iron deficiency is no more likely to occur in vegetarians than nonvegetarians. In fact, children diagnosed with anemia are often told to consume more fruits and vegetables, not only because they contain iron, but also because the vitamin C increases iron absorption from other foods.

So how can a child get enough iron so that this depletion never occurs? Not how you might think.

Only about one-fifth of iron in a standard diet comes from meat. Animal flesh of all kinds provides iron but not in quantities significant enough to deem it the best or only quality source.

The same is true for dairy. Dairy products are deficient in iron unless they are enriched, but even then the iron is not well absorbed. Cow's milk is so low in iron that you'd have to drink 50 gallons to get the iron found in a single bowl of spinach. Furthermore, if you consume too many dairy products, there is a greater possibility of iron deficiency since they actually tend to block the absorption of iron in the body. The addition of modest amounts of milk or cheese to a meat meal has been shown to reduce iron absorption by 50 to 60 percent.

An abundance of iron is found in dried beans, dark-green leafy vegetables, and whole grains. Raisins, watermelon, and blackstrap molasses are also good sources of iron and better per calorie than meat. Apricots and whole-grain or iron-fortified breads also provide iron, as do iron-fortified cereals—without the cholesterol and extra fat you'd ingest from meat. Other foods that contain iron include almonds, avocados, beets, dates, kelp, lentils, millet, parsley, peaches, pears, prunes, pumpkins, rice, wheat bran, and sesame seeds.

Values of Some High-Iron-Content Foods

Item	Serving	Calories	Fat	Protein	Iron
Kidney beans	1 cup	612	1.5 g	43 g	15 mg
Lima beans	1 cup	601	1 g	38 g	13 mg
Chickpeas	1 cup	728	12 g	38.5 g	12.5 mg
Spinach	1 bunch	75	1 g	9.5 g	9 mg
Soybeans	1 cup	376	17 g	33 g	9 mg
Broccoli	1 bunch	170	2 g	18 g	5 mg
Cabbage	1 med head	227	2.5 g	13 g	5 mg

Source: USDA—Nutrient Data Lab (Sept. 1996). All data are based on raw vegetables.

Also, remember that iron absorption increases if a food high in vitamin C is present in the meal. For example, to get this enhanced absorption, one might eat a salad made with garbanzo beans, peas, and spinach (good sources of iron) combined with tomatoes and peppers (good sources of vitamin C). Brown rice and tofu served with vitamin C foods such as tomato sauce and broccoli can double or triple your iron absorption. For a high-iron breakfast, try adding a few nuts, dried fruits, or seeds to your iron-fortified cereal. You can also drink a glass of orange juice to ensure the extra absorption.

If you are still concerned about the adequacy of your child's iron intake, you can always provide supplements. There are many varieties available, in both tablet and liquid form. Some people are concerned that iron supplements lead to problems such as constipation. If it occurs, try brands in which the iron source is natural, not synthetic. Speak with the nutritional consultant at your natural food store about iron supplements derived from plants and herbs.

Remember that iron deficiency is common among kids and teens of all eating persuasions. The most important thing is that, whatever their eating patterns are, you ensure your child's diet contains plenty of iron-rich foods.

But My Child Is an Athlete!

There's nothing like the feeling of victory when your child runs across the finish line or scores the winning goal. Although you vow to remain the even-tempered parent who would *never* think to scream at the referee for his obvious blindness and prejudice against your child, you can't help but be invested in her competitive success. That is why a few nights before the big game you find yourself in the meat aisle hearing your own mother's voice in your head — "Meat equals strength, meat equals strength, meat equals strength" — and reaching for the juiciest rib eye you can find. It's also why you give in to your child's pleas for those mega-man protein supplements even though you've heard the concerns about their usefulness—and safety.

Although your young athlete's protein needs may be elevated because training increases amino acid metabolism, vegetarian diets can meet caloric needs and include good sources of protein, such as beans and soy products, and you won't need special foods or supplements. The US Olympic Committee on Vegetarian Diets agrees: "If care is taken to include a wide variety of foods, vegetarian diets can be nutritionally adequate to support athletic performance." Moreover, "Whether an individual is a recreational or world-class athlete, being a vegetarian does not diminish natural talent or athletic performance. As far back as the Ancient Games, Greek athletes trained on vegetarian diets and displayed amazing ability in competitive athletics."

Many well-known athletes swear by plant-based eating. Dave Scott, recognized as the greatest triathlete in the world, is a six-time winner of the Iron Man Triathlon, breaking his own record three consecutive years. He calls the idea that people, and especially athletes, need animal protein a "ridiculous fallacy." Many people consider vegetarian Dave Scott the fittest man who ever lived.

Another devout vegetarian triathlete, Sixto Linares, says that he was a vegetarian for over 14 years before his parents finally began to accept that the diet might be good for him. During that time, he broke the world record for the one-day triathlon by swimming 4.8 miles, cycling 185 miles, and then running 52.4 miles.

Carl Lewis, seven-time Olympic gold-medal sprinter, trains and competes while eating a solely plant-based diet. Bill Pearl, who won the Mr. Universe title four times, last when he was 41 years old, is a perfect example of meatless muscle.

And, though not a world-class athlete, my own daughter, Deanna, is a perfect example of a teenage athlete who happens to be a vegetarian. She's not a fanatic and has no problem occasionally indulging in her grandma's spaghetti with turkey sauce or cornflake chicken, but her diet has been primarily vegetarian since birth. Yet she is not only the starting pitcher on her high school softball team but works out rigorously at the gym for an hour and a half five days a week. She has incredible physical strength and stamina, and as far as I can remember she's been ill only a handful of days in her life and has missed only three or four days of school in the past 11 years because of illness. Furthermore, she has never taken an antibiotic in her life — she's never been sick enough to need one.

Other Famous Vegetarian Athletes

Pat Reeves
   *Britain's female power-lifting champion eight
   consecutive years*
Estelle Gray and Cheryl Marek
   World record holders for cross-country tandem cycling
Hank Aaron
   Record holder for career home runs
Sally Eastall
   Marathon runner

Cory Everson
Bodybuilder, six-time Ms Olympia
Di Edwards
Runner, Olympic semifinalist
Martina Navratilova
International tennis champion
Ridgely Abele, fifth-degree black belt
US Karate Association grand champion
Edwin Moses
Olympic gold-medal hurdler
Joe Namath
Legendary Super Bowl champion
Jack LaLaine
Fitness and exercise guru
Andreas Cahling
Bodybuilder, Mr. International
Billy Jean King
Legendary tennis champion
Bill Walton
All-star center and NBA champion
Desmond Howard
Heisman Trophy winner
Daniel Poneman
Future "Hall of Famer"

The achievements of these and other athletes, although they do not prove that a vegetarian diet is superior, set a precedent for outstanding health, strength, and competitive advantage for those athletes who have chosen vegetarian diets.

The Reality:
A Vegetarian Diet Is Healthy for Young People

Like all children, vegetarians need enough food variety and energy—in the form of calories—to fuel their growth and fulfill their nutrient needs. The years between 13 and 19 are full of rapid changes, so nutritional needs are notably high during this period. A vegetarian diet can be more than adequate to support these needs.

Yet such a diet, like any other, can be unhealthful. You need to strive for balance. Just as you would be concerned if your child ate only cheeseburgers and hot dogs, so too you should be concerned if your child eats only potato chips and french fries or, for that matter, only carrots and apples.

As I mentioned earlier, the ADA declares that an appropriately planned vegetarian diet can provide adequate nutrition and prevent osteoporosis, kidney disease, diabetes, and some types of cancer, such as lung, colorectal, and breast. Vegetarian diets offer these disease-protection benefits because of their lower amounts of saturated fat, cholesterol, and animal protein and higher concentrations of folate and antioxidants—such as vitamins C and E. Vegetarian diets have also been used successfully in weight reduction in obese children and adolescents.

A major proponent of a vegetarian diet is Dr. Nathan Pritikin, author of *The Pritikin Diet* and recognized expert on nutrition, who recommends it as part of a comprehensive health program to prevent and even reverse coronary artery disease. And if you think you don't have to worry about coronary disease in children, tell that to my friend whose 21-year-old son dropped dead on the basketball court last year—cause of death: arteriosclerosis.

The shocking truth is that autopsies done on accident victims as young as 12 often indicate fatty streaks in the arteries similar to those of 50–60 year olds of previous generations, whose intake of saturated fat was far less than it is today. Research has shown that the number of deaths from coronary artery disease is significantly lower in vegetarians than in nonvegetarians and that a vegetarian diet can dramatically reduce the possibility of heart attack and stroke.

If you still have doubts, do your own research until you really understand the facts about vegetarian eating. There are many resources available, several of which are listed in the appendix.

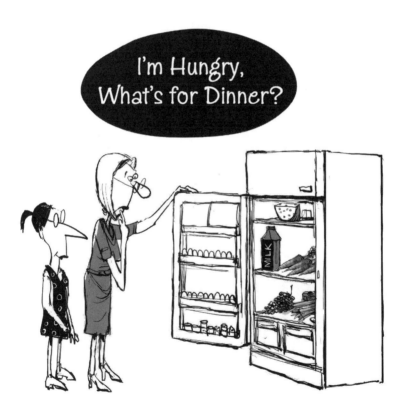

CHAPTER 3

I'm Hungry,
What's for Dinner?

**From Grocery Store to Table for
the Harried House Parent**

My mom, bless her heart, is 85 years old and still going strong. One of her favorite pastimes is looking through cookbooks and the newspaper's food section for vegetarian recipes for meals she can make for my family and me.

I love and appreciate her desire to cook special foods for us so that we can feel as nourished in her home as those who eat her brisket of beef or famous veal Parmesan (which used to be my favorite). But the truth is most vegetarians prefer to eat very simply, and it seems that, the longer people are vegetarians, the simpler their tastes become.

When I announced my vegetarian intentions in 1970, I tried to tell my mom that I'd be happy with steamed vegetables, a bowl of rice, and a side of beans, but when you try to tell a Jewish mother to give her child just rice and beans it does not compute. Simple meals are not in a Jewish mother's universe.

Furthermore, in 1970 there were only about three vegetarian cookbooks on the bookstore shelves and one tiny natural food store a half hour away from our house. There was nothing that came close to resembling a Whole Foods or Wild Oats Market. Needless to say, our local supermarket did not have the now common natural food section. The words *tofu* and *veggie burger* were not part of anybody's everyday vocabulary—at least not in the suburbs of Chicago—and there was my poor mother trying to figure out what to do. In retrospect, I realize I didn't give her enough credit for what she had to go through to accommodate my lifestyle.

But, although she didn't have access to the abundance of options and tools available today, times were simpler then, and she was a stay-at-home mom. The moms and dads of today juggle not only their own demanding careers and activities but also more baseball, soccer, hockey, skating, football, volleyball, karate, skiing, drama, music lessons, scouting, and wall-climbing than our parents knew existed in 1970! With all those responsibilities, abundant resources or not, who has time to learn how to prepare vegetable flambé?

Our Simple Approach: RTM (Replace the Meat!)

This chapter is written for those parents who are in a position to do only the required minimum. For whatever reason, and I know there are many, you're not able to add more than 10 minutes a meal to accommodate your vegetarian. You're willing to learn a few new recipes and ways to cook for your child, and are even willing to learn the difference between tofu and tempeh, but are not able to make this into a huge undertaking.

Whenever possible, you'd like to continue cooking for your family the way you always have, and believe it or not, and as my mother discovered, in most cases you can. With simple substitutions for the meat portion of the meal, your vegetarian child will be both nourished and satisfied.

For example, you can make easy tacos or burritos with vegetarian refried beans instead of meat. Or, if you're making Chinese food, when it's time to add the meat, add tofu to your vegetarian's portion instead.

The most common meat substitutes, besides beans, are called tofu, tempeh, seitan, and TVP. If you can learn about these four basic ingredients, you're practically home free!

Common Meat Substitutes

Tofu *(TOE-foo)*, also known as soybean curd, is a versatile food made by curdling hot soy milk. It's an excellent source of high-quality protein that contains all nine amino acids. It's low in saturated fat and contains no cholesterol. With a custard-like consistency, tofu acts like a sponge in recipes, absorbing flavors from other ingredients. Tofu is usually found in the produce section, although some stores sell tofu in the dairy or deli section. There are four different types of tofu that vary by firmness and texture.

- **EXTRA FIRM TOFU** contains little water and maintains its shape well, making it ideal for slicing, dicing, frying, and broiling.
- **FIRM TOFU** is not as dense, although it also holds its shape for slicing, dicing, and frying. It works well as a cheese substitute in recipes calling for cottage, ricotta, or even cream cheese.

◆ **SOFT TOFU** is much less dense and is often used to reduce or replace eggs. It can also be blended to replace sour cream or yogurt.

◆ **SILKEN TOFU** has a much finer consistency, almost liquid, and is ideal for blending into dressings and sauces.

Seitan *(SAY-tan)* is a flavored form of wheat gluten, made from whole-wheat flour mixed with water and kneaded. It has a chewy consistency and is a good replacement for poultry or beef in stir-fries or stews. Seitan is a high-protein, low-fat, no-cholesterol food usually found in the refrigerated section of the grocery store. It typically comes in small tubs, like margarine, or in shrink-wrapped plastic. Seitan is best steamed or sautéed in a little oil. If you bake seitan, be sure not to overbake it — it gets dense when it loses its moisture.

Tempeh *(TEM-pay)* is a cultured soybean cake. Its tender, chewy consistency makes it a versatile meat substitute. Tempeh can be grilled, deep-fried, sautéed, steamed, baked, or micro-waved and holds its shape well. It is an excellent source of high-quality, cholesterol-free protein that contains all nine essential amino acids. It's also a good source of dietary fiber, calcium, B vitamins, and iron. Tempeh is found in the frozen food or refrigerated section of natural food stores. Frozen, packaged tempeh will stay fresh for up to a year. Once thawed and opened, it will stay fresh in the refrigerator for about one month. Because it is a cultured product, a white culture is normal and does not indicate spoilage.

TVP, or texturized vegetable protein, is made from soybeans. TVP usually comes in a dried form and must be reconstituted in water. It is available in many different sizes and shapes, from powder to chunks, and in flavors such as beef and chicken. It is especially good for replacing ground meats and can be found in the bulk section of your natural food store.

Different Kinds of Vegetarians

Before you switch to soy milk, first determine the type of vegetarian your child has chosen to become. It makes a big difference if your child wants to be a vegan as opposed to a semi-vegetarian. Where in the spectrum does your child fall?

What Type of Vegetarian Is Your Child?

 Vegan or pure vegetarian

What They **Do** Eat
- Anything not derived from animal sources

What They **Don't** Eat
- All meat and any foods that come from an animal, including eggs and dairy

 Lacto-ovo vegetarian

What They **Do** Eat
- Same as above, with the addition of eggs and dairy

What They **Don't** Eat
- Any form of meat, fish, or poultry

Semivegetarian

What They **Do** Eat

- Same as above, with the addition of fish or poultry

What They **Don't** Eat

- Any form of red meat, including beef, pork, veal, or lamb

Now that you understand which type of vegetarianism your child has chosen, and are familiar with the "big four" meat substitutes, you are prepared to go to the grocery store and buy the right foods to make cooking and snack time a breeze. The shopping lists and cooking suggestions that follow are illustrated with icons to lead you directly to the information pertinent to your child.

Replace the Meat — BREAKFAST

If you're having: Scrambled eggs/omelettes
Leave out: Eggs

Replace with: Tofu: buy firm or soft tofu, mash it, plop it in the skillet, and sauté it with salt and oil — add veggies such as mushrooms, spinach, tomatoes, etc.

Replace with: You can use eggs but may still want to use tofu for health benefits.

If you're having: Bacon or sausages

Leave out: Pork or beef

 Replace with: Soy bacon or sausages

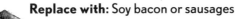 **Replace with:** Turkey bacon or sausages

If you're having: Waffles or pancakes

Leave out: Eggs

Replace with: One of many egg substitutes; refer to the egg-substitution list that follows for suggestions

 Vegan note: Be sure that your waffle or pancake mix doesn't contain any hidden dairy products.

If you're having: Cereal and milk

Leave out: Milk

Replace with: Soy milk or rice milk

If you're having: Yogurt with granola and fruit

Leave out: Dairy yogurt

Replace with: Soy yogurt

If you're having: Oatmeal or other hot cereal

Leave out: Milk and butter

Replace with: Soy or rice milk and margarine

If you're having: Toast or bagels

Leave out: Cream cheese and butter

    Replace with: Apple butter, pure fruit jams, tahini, soy cream cheese

Common Egg Substitutes

- A popular egg substitute is Ener-G Egg Replacer, made from potato starch, tapioca flour, leavening agents, and a gum derived from cottonseed. It's meant to replace the leavening/binding characteristics of eggs in baking but can be used for non-baked foods and quiches too. This product can be found in your natural food store. Just follow the directions on the box.
- Try using two ounces of soft tofu, blended with a little water. This mixture can be substituted for an egg to add consistency. Or try the same quantity of mashed beans, mashed potatoes, or nut butters.
- Mashed bananas make excellent egg substitutes. Half a mashed banana roughly equals one egg.
- Applesauce or puréed fruit can also be used as a flavorful substitute. A mere quarter cup of applesauce equals one egg.
- Try one teaspoon of soy flour plus one tablespoon of water to substitute for one egg.
- Two tablespoons of water plus one tablespoon of oil and two teaspoons of baking powder equal one whole egg.

Replace the Meat — LUNCH

If you're having: Simplest sandwich

Leave out: Meat

 Replace with: Cheese, green peppers, sprouts, lettuce, tomatoes, cucumbers, onions, avocado, and any soy or wheat luncheon meat on whole-grain bread

If you're having: BLT

Leave out: Bacon

 Replace with: Turkey

Vegan note: There are many excellent varieties of soy bacon.

If you're having: Grilled cheese

Leave out: Cheese

Replace with: Soy or veggie cheese

If you're having: Sloppy Joes

Leave out: Meat

 Replace with: Ground turkey

Vegan note: Use mashed firm tofu, or TVP granules.

If you're having: "Gourmet" sandwiches
Leave out: Meat

Replace with: Sautéed peppers, zucchinis, mushrooms, or sliced tomatoes, or slice extra firm tofu half an inch thick and drain, marinate in vinaigrette, and then sauté in oil. Add fresh mozzarella or a slice of Monterey Jack, fresh basil, and Italian dressing on French bread

Vegan note: Leave out the cheese, or use a soy or veggie cheese substitute.

If you're having: Chef's salad
Leave out: Chef's salad meat

Replace with: Garbanzo or kidney beans (canned), raisins, walnuts, feta or hard cheeses, and mandarin oranges

Vegan note: Leave out the cheese, or use a soy or veggie cheese substitute.

If you're having: Soup
Leave out: Meat or meat base

Replace with: Any soup, home cooked or canned. Be sure it's not made from a meat base. There are over 20 different varieties of vegetable-based soups

at the natural food store, including instant soups in
a cup

Vegan note: Watch out for chowders and creamy
soups that contain dairy!

Replace the Meat — DINNER

American night
If you're having: Hot dogs, hamburgers, baked beans
Leave out: Beef hot dogs and hamburgers

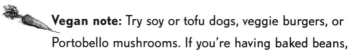**Replace with:** Turkey dogs, turkey burgers, even
turkey and chicken bratwursts (don't forget the
French fries)

Vegan note: Try soy or tofu dogs, veggie burgers, or
Portobello mushrooms. If you're having baked beans,
choose the vegetarian variety.

Italian night
If you're having: Lasagna, spaghetti, eggplant Parmesan, etc.
Leave out: Ground beef and meat sauce

Replace with: Equal amounts of ground turkey and
chopped carrots, zucchini, and mushrooms in marinara sauce

Vegan note: Try buying veggie meatballs frozen or in a mix. Beware of hidden cheeses, especially if you use store-bought pasta sauce.

Mexican night
If you're having: Tacos, burritos, tostados, enchiladas
Leave out: Ground beef
 Replace with: Chicken or ground turkey

 Replace with: Vegetarian refried beans, rice, or sautéed vegetables; add your favorite cheese

 Vegan note: Watch out for dairy in Mexican dishes and lard in many refried beans.

If you're having: Chili
Leave out: Ground beef
 Replace with: Ground turkey

 Vegan note: Use TVP, extra beans, and veggies.

French night
If you're having: Quiche
Leave out: Ham
 Replace with: Vegetables such as spinach, zucchini, broccoli, or mushrooms; you can also try "fake" ham made from soy or wheat

Any stew or stir-fry
If you're having: Beef Stroganoff, beef stew, Mulligan stew
Leave out: Meat
    Replace with: Seitan or tempeh

Meat-and-potatoes night
If you're having: Steak, lamb, veal, chicken, fish
Leave out: Meat portion
    Replace with: Sliced and sautéed tofu, sautéed
        tempeh or seitan, or any type of beans

If these simple suggestions don't even fit your idea of a realistic daily schedule, the frozen food aisle of your local natural food market is brimming with everything from tofu pot pie to pasta primavera and just about any ethnic cuisine you can imagine from Pad Thai to spinach-and-feta pockets, from vegetable curry to pizzas overflowing with fabulous-looking veggies and goat cheese.

And on those nights when you're fresh out of tempeh and the freezer is bare, and you have time to cook only for the rest of the family, just leave out the meat and give them the trimmings. A salad, a baked potato, and a big serving of lightly steamed vegetables are more than adequate, and the food pyramid police will give you less of a citation than if you order a pizza.

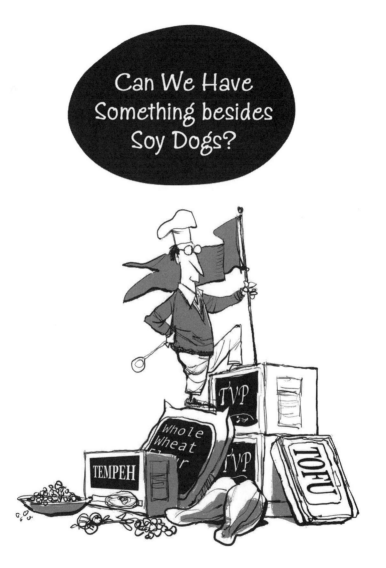

CHAPTER 4

Can We Have Something besides Soy Dogs?

Emily's Recipes for the Adventurous Chef

If you thought you loved to cook steaks, let me tell you vegetarian cooking is a joy! The options are endless, the colors are vibrant, and the cleanup is a breeze. If you think you are in store for bulgur loafs and oatmeal pancakes, think again. This chapter is full of vegetarian recipes bursting with flavor and pizzazz.

My intention here isn't to provide you with a complete cookbook, since the bookstore shelves are already lined with titles ranging from *The Giant Book of Tofu* to *The Voluptuous Vegan*. In fact, on Amazon.com, there are 1,269 books listed under the category "vegetarian cooking." My goal is to give you some exciting recipes beyond tofu dogs and "substitution" dishes that will introduce you to a new world of vegetarian delicacies.

These recipes have been inspired by the finest cuisines of the world, among them Mediterranean, Middle Eastern, Indian, American, and Far Eastern. They mix flavors, textures, and colors to create exceptional, nutritionally balanced recipes, featuring vegan and light dairy alternatives to animal proteins.

Actually, this chapter could be subtitled "Meatless Dishes Even Meat Eaters Will Love" since the recipes show you how mouthwatering vegetarian cooking can be. In fact, I serve them to my meat-eating friends and relatives all the time, and they don't run screaming from the room—they ask for the recipes. Not only are all of these recipes vegetarian, but in many cases they are also more healthful and lower in fat than their mainstream counterparts. You don't have to be a vegetarian to enjoy this food any more than you need to be Italian to enjoy lasagna!

And for those of you with a little Martha Stewart in your genes, these recipes are even appropriate for a social setting. These foods don't broadcast "vegetarian" to the world. Like you, I prefer to use mealtime with friends and family for socializing, not moralizing.

I hope your family and friends enjoy these recipes as much as mine do.

A beloved master was asked by his students,

"What is the best food to eat for our spiritual growth?"

To which he replied: "The food your mother makes you."

Breakfast — A Healthy Start for Your Child

Although breakfast is often referred to as the most important meal of the day, many children and teens consistently skip it. According to the American Dietetic Association, one out of six fifth graders doesn't eat breakfast, and the numbers get more grim as children get older. Although breakfast consumption has declined in all age groups over the past 25 years, the worst offenders are female adolescents aged 15–18. Sound like your child? In the mad morning rush to get ready for school and work, the whole family may be tempted to skip breakfast. Please don't!

Studies show that habitual breakfast skippers have less energy to participate in morning activities, are more likely to feel tired, and find it more difficult to concentrate and learn. A recent Harvard study showed that children who don't eat breakfast are more often tardy and absent from school than those who do. Unfortunately, these breakfast skippers are unlikely to make up for nutrients missed at breakfast later in the day even though they often end up overeating at lunch and dinner.

Conversely, children who eat a healthy breakfast are more alert, creative, and energetic. The same Harvard study shows that they perform better on school tests. It is also reported that adolescents who consume breakfast tend to make more appropriate food choices throughout the day. A study done at the Children's Nutrition Research Center (CNRC) found that sufficient intake of vitamins and minerals, such as zinc and calcium, as well as protein and carbohydrates, is much higher among adolescents who eat breakfast (see www.ars.usda.gov/is/pr/2002/020621.htm).

Eating breakfast is more than just a good habit; it's a key part of achieving maximum nutrition. While your vegetarian child will be content with a simple breakfast such as scrambled tofu and veggie bacon or just a bowl of cereal and soy milk with a glass of orange juice, these more adventurous recipes will broaden your options. Not only are they delicious, but most are also packed with vitamins, minerals, and protein.

Mmmmm Morning Muffins (*Makes 12*)

Typical muffins are laden with fat and sugar. These are different
—each hearty muffin is full of protein, fiber, vitamins, and minerals, plus omega-3 essential fatty acids from the walnuts and
flaxseeds. Store them in individual plastic bags for an easy snack
or an energy boost after soccer practice.

Ingredients
1 cup whole-wheat flour
1 cup unbleached white flour
1/2 cup soy protein powder
2 tsp baking powder
1 tsp baking soda
1 tsp cinnamon
2 large ripe bananas
3/4 cup fortified soy milk
1/4 cup vegetable oil
1/4 cup blackstrap molasses
1/4 cup maple syrup
2 tsp apple cider vinegar
1 cup raisins
1 cup dried cranberries
1 cup sweetened flaked coconut
1 tbsp ground flaxseeds
1/2 cup chopped walnuts

Directions

1. Preheat oven to 350 degrees. Lightly oil a 12-count muffin tin.

2. In a large bowl, combine flours, protein powder, baking powder, baking soda, and cinnamon. Stir dry mixture until ingredients are evenly dispersed.

3. In a smaller bowl, mash bananas. Stir in soy milk, oil, blackstrap molasses, maple syrup, and apple cider vinegar.

4. Add wet mixture to dry ingredients, stirring just until blended. Stir in raisins, cranberries, coconut, ground flaxseeds, and walnuts.

5. Fill muffin cups and bake for about 30 minutes, until muffins pull away from the sides of the tin and spring back when you press the tops lightly.

 TIP: Every major grocery store now carries flaxseeds. If you can only find them whole, don't worry, just grind them yourself in a food processor or coffee bean grinder. Grinding the flaxseeds enables their nutrients to be more readily absorbed. Blackstrap molasses comes from the third and final extraction of sugar refining. It contains lower sugar content than other sweeteners and is the highest in quantities of vitamins and minerals of all molasses varieties. Also, be sure to use real maple syrup, not the popular sugar-laden or artificially sweetened varieties.

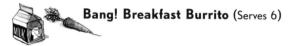 **Bang! Breakfast Burrito** (Serves 6)

In my family, breakfast burritos were a Sunday treat. This simple recipe uses tofu instead of eggs, and the result is love at first bite. Remember, any vegetable can be substituted for the ones listed. And, when you have leftover baked potatoes, this is a great way not to let them go to waste!

Ingredients
2–3 tbsp extra-virgin olive oil
1 red bell pepper, chopped
1 green pepper, chopped
1 tsp ground cumin
1/2 tsp ground coriander
1 lb firm tofu, crumbled
3–4 baked potatoes, cubed
1/4 cup chopped cilantro
Whole-wheat tortillas
Fresh or bottled salsa
Jalapeno pepper (optional)
Grated cheese or soy cheese (optional)

Directions
1. Heat oil in a 10-inch skillet over medium heat.
2. Add peppers, cumin, and coriander. Sauté until vegetables are soft.
3. Crumble tofu into skillet with vegetables and stir.
4. Add cubed potatoes and cilantro and stir. Sauté approximately 10 minutes.

5. To assemble burritos, place a third of a cup of the filling mixture in a whole-wheat tortilla, roll it up, and top it with salsa. Serve warm, topped with cheese if desired.

 TIP: These burritos are delicious topped with cheese and can make a satisfying lunch or after-school snack! Make a large batch and freeze the burritos individually in aluminum foil. They are excellent when reheated in the oven for 20–30 minutes at 350 degrees. For those who don't have the time to cube whole potatoes, you can always use frozen hash browns instead.

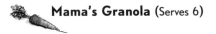 **Mama's Granola** (Serves 6)

Children love granola, but so many of the store-bought kinds are high in sugar and fat. This tasty recipe is low fat and delicious.

Ingredients
3 cups rolled oats
1 cup sweetened cornflakes
1/2 cup toasted wheat germ
1/2 cup chopped almonds (optional)
1 tsp ground cinnamon
1/2 tsp grated nutmeg
1/2 tsp salt
1/2 cup thawed apple juice concentrate
1/2 cup maple syrup
1 tsp vanilla extract
1 1/2 cups dried fruit (raisins, cranberries, bananas, apricots, etc.)

Directions

1. Preheat oven to 300 degrees. Coat two baking sheets with vegetable oil cooking spray and set aside.
2. Place oats in a colander and dampen with cold water. Transfer to a medium-sized mixing bowl. Add cereal flakes, wheat germ, almonds, cinnamon, nutmeg, and salt and stir until mixed.
3. In a small bowl, combine juice, syrup, and vanilla. Pour over oat mixture and stir until evenly coated. Spread granola mixture in prepared pans. Bake at 300 degrees until golden brown, about 30–35 minutes, turning every 10 minutes so that it browns evenly.
4. Stir in your favorite combination of dried fruits and bake five minutes more. Let cool thoroughly and store in an airtight container until ready to use.

 TIP: This recipe works well with dried cranberries and is awesome in the morning with soy milk. Or you can pack some for a snack in plastic bags to keep the kids going all afternoon.

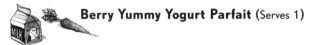

Berry Yummy Yogurt Parfait (Serves 1)

What child wouldn't like dessert for breakfast? Don't let this scrumptious, indulgent treat deceive you; it's packed with goodness for your kids. Interpret this recipe loosely, substituting different flavors and fruits depending on what's in season or in your refrigerator.

Ingredients
3/4 cup low-fat vanilla yogurt or soy yogurt

2 tbsp honey

1/4 tsp vanilla

1/2 cup Mama's Granola or any healthy cereal

1/2 cup blueberries, strawberries, raspberries, or other fruit

Directions
1. In a small bowl, blend yogurt, honey, and vanilla (or just use already sweetened yogurt—staying away from any sweetened with aspartame).
2. Using a tall glass (or a large wine goblet), layer about a third of the granola on the bottom, top with about a third of the yogurt mixture, and then add a third of the berries.
3. Repeat layers twice. Serve with a long spoon.

 TIP: Consider using blueberries, which are extremely high in antioxidants.

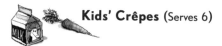 **Kids' Crêpes** (Serves 6)

Crêpes make a wonderful disguise for healthy fruits and vegetables of all kinds. There are many excellent crêpe recipes, but this one is simple and vegan.

Ingredients
1/3 cup whole-wheat pastry flour
2/3 cup soy milk

Filling Ideas
Bananas, strawberries, or other fruit
Soft cream cheese mixed with a little honey

Directions
1. Blend flour and soy milk in a food processor and let sit for five minutes. Meanwhile, heat a non-stick skillet until very hot. You shouldn't need to use any oil.
2. Reblend the batter and pour onto the heated skillet with one hand while moving the skillet in a circular motion with the other to coat the entire bottom. Pour any remaining batter back into the food processor.
3. Heat until the edges shrink in and you can loosen the side of the crêpe with a spatula. Either with a flick of the wrist (for seasoned crêpe makers) or by sliding the crêpe onto a plate, then flipping it back into the pan, cook the other side for several seconds, but not as long as the first side.

4. Stack the cooked crêpes on top of each other on a plate in a warm oven until the rest are made. Remember to quickly pulse the batter before each crêpe because some settling will occur.
5. Precut all fruit into small pieces and set in bowls. When the kids are ready to eat, they can add as much and as many types of fruit as they want.

Remember to fill the crêpes with the most beautiful side down so that it will be visible when rolled.

 TIP: Crêpes are a versatile treat that can be enjoyed any time of the day. Experiment with the fillings your family likes best. Crêpes can be enjoyed as appetizers stuffed with mushrooms and cheese, tomato and spinach, or feta and olive. Snack crêpes can be prepared with light fillings such as blueberry jam, cinnamon apples, or chocolate. For meal-sized crêpes, just go extra heavy on the stuffing with cheese, veggies, and tofu. Crêpes make excellent desserts filled or topped with ice cream, pudding, or even honey, cinnamon, and a dash of lemon juice.

Lunch — What?! No Snickers?!

Think back to the days of school cafeteria lunches. Do images of "mystery meat" haunt your mind? In retrospect, I see that the food-service director did the best she could to plan healthy, well-balanced lunches. Usually, however, there was meat in the main course, so school lunches were never an option for me. And many parents just can't bring themselves to let their kids eat a greasy grilled cheese sandwich on white bread, genetically modified chips, sugar-drenched canned pears with an expiration date in the next century, and a carton of bovine growth hormone-laden milk.

 Be sure to swap the white bread for a nourishing whole grain variety.

Although the variety of foods offered by many schools has improved, there still may not be many options for your vegetarian child. More often than not, a packed lunch is the most healthful option. Kids in junior high and high school get to choose from a wide variety of tempting foods at the school buffet lunch line—but you may still want to pack their lunches.

 Good old P. B. and J. is always a hit with vegetarians. Try adding sliced bananas or chopped dates.

Or teens may want to pack their own lunches, so it's a good idea to have a wide variety of vegetarian selections on hand. If the choices aren't varied, appealing, or *there*, your child will find it easier to take money and resort to pizza — about the only vegetarian dish available in most cafeterias. As a parent, it's your job to help your children get into the habit of thinking about nutritious vegetarian lunches, since lunch is the meal that will sustain them through their afternoon activities.

 Debra's daughter's favorite lunch is salad in a bag. She takes a big Ziploc, puts in lots of lettuce, carrots, cucumbers, celery and green peppers, then adds her favorite dressing in a corner of the bag and when she's ready to eat she shakes it up!

The following recipes work well at home but can also work in a lunch box. If you're like every mother and worry about anything made with unrefrigerated mayonnaise, then freeze the juice box the night before, and it will keep the lunch cool like an ice pack and will be defrosted enough to drink by lunchtime.

Curly Q "Tuna" Salad (Serves 6)

This rendition of a tuna pasta salad is high in protein and great in taste. The recipe doubles easily and keeps well.

Ingredients
1 pkg curly Q pasta
1 pkg baked marinated tofu (any flavor), finely diced
2 stalks celery, finely diced
1 red pepper, cubed
1/2 cup soy mayonnaise
1/2 tsp salt
1/2 tsp freshly ground pepper

Directions
1. Bring a large pot of lightly salted water to a boil. Add pasta and cook according to package directions. Drain, rinse under cold running water until cool, and then drain again. Transfer to large serving bowl.
2. Add remaining ingredients and toss gently to combine. Serve right away or cover and chill until needed.

TIP: Soy mayonnaise is readily available in natural food stores. A popular brand is Nayonnaise.

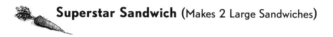 **Superstar Sandwich** (Makes 2 Large Sandwiches)

Here's a sandwich that provides 68 percent of a woman's recommended protein for the day and over 50 percent of a man's recommended protein. Make the sandwich with one type of veggie meat or use several types.

Ingredients
3/4 cup shelled green soybeans (edamame)
1 tbsp Dijon mustard
1/2 tsp garlic powder
Salt to taste
2 large Kaiser rolls, whole-wheat sandwich buns,
    or other hearty bread
8 slices veggie meat
Thinly sliced tomato and cucumber
Spinach or lettuce leaves

Directions
1. Cook soybeans for five minutes over high heat in boiling water.
2. Drain beans, reserving cooking water in a blender or food processor.

3. Combine beans, mustard, garlic powder, and salt. Purée until smooth, adding more water if it appears too thick to spread.

4. Halve the rolls and slather each half with soybean purée. On the bottom half of each bun, arrange half of the veggie meat slices, tomato slices, cucumbers, and spinach or lettuce. Spread bun tops with remaining purée.

5. Place tops on sandwiches and wrap tightly in plastic wrap or parchment paper. Slice sandwiches in half right through wrapper for easy eating.

Simple Hummus Surprise (Serves 1)

Ingredients

2 slices multigrain bread

2 tbsp hummus of choice

Assorted sliced or diced veggies such as carrots, tomatoes, cucumbers, peppers

Other things such as olives, capers, basil, beans, onions, pickles

Whatever . . . be creative!

Directions

1. Spread hummus on bread.

2. Top with whatever sounds good or looks good to your child—several things together taste delicious!

TIP: You'll enjoy coming up with new variations of this. There are some great hummus flavors out now—roasted red pepper, garlic, and herb—and you can even find them at the local supermarket. They also make excellent dips for veggie platters, or pack the hummus in a container with cut-up veggies for your child's lunch.

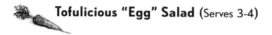

Tofulicious "Egg" Salad (Serves 3-4)

Ingredients
1 pkg extra firm tofu

3 tbsp soy mayonnaise

2 tbsp dill pickle relish

1 stalk celery, minced

1 tbsp minced onion

1 tbsp Dijon mustard

1 tsp turmeric

1/4 cup slivered almonds

1/2 cup plump raisins

Salt and pepper to taste

Directions
1. Break tofu into large pieces and press water out in a paper towel. Crumble into bowl.
2. Add all ingredients to tofu and mix thoroughly. Add more soy mayonnaise, if desired, to reach preferred consistency.
3. Serve on toasted bread with melted cheese, sliced tomato, and crispy Romaine lettuce.

TIP: This salad tastes even better the next day, after it has marinated. If you like it saltier, you can add one tablespoon of tamari to the mixture.

Not Your Average "Chicken" Fingers (Serves 4-6)

This recipe is especially for those tired of eating mushy tofu. Kids love these firm and chewy breaded nuggets, as will your nonvegetarian friends and family. If you freeze your tofu, it will be firm enough to be breaded without falling apart. Try putting a few squares in a freezer bag and then defrosting them in a bowl of warm water when needed. They take only a few minutes to defrost and are great when you need to get lunch or dinner on the table fast.

Ingredients
2 pkg extra firm tofu, defrosted and well drained
1/2 cup unsweetened soy milk
1 heaping tbsp poultry seasoning
Garlic powder
1 tsp seasoned salt
Pepper
1/2 cup bread crumbs
3 tbsp wheat germ
2 tbsp yellow cornmeal
1/2 cup flour

Directions

1. Preheat oven to 400 degrees. Lightly oil non-stick baking sheet.
2. Cut defrosted tofu in slices about half an inch thick and squeeze as much moisture as you can out of them with a paper towel.
3. In a bowl, whisk together soy milk, poultry seasoning, garlic powder, seasoned salt, and pepper to taste. Don't be shy with the poultry seasoning. In another bowl, combine bread crumbs, wheat germ, and corn-meal. Put your flour in a third bowl.
4. Dip the tofu slices into the flour and then into the soy milk and spices mixture. Finally, coat each tofu slice with the bread crumbs mixture.
5. You can either fry your "chicken fingers" in a little oil or spray a baking sheet with non-stick spray and bake at 400 until lightly golden on both sides.

 TIP: Serve hot with ketchup, barbecue sauce, or marinara sauce for dipping.

The Packed Lunch

There's definitely an art to preparing a healthy packed vegetarian lunch, but saying bye-bye to Twinkies and Lunchables won't be so hard with these simple tips. All you have to do is add two or three of the following kid-preferred foods to one of the above "main courses" and you have a complete meal:

+ a soup-sized thermos filled with some hearty veggie soup—probably left over from the night before;
+ a small bag of lightly salted "half the oil" potato chips, yellow or blue corn tortilla chips, veggie chips, or mini rice cakes;
+ dried fruit (raisins, apricots, cherries), nuts, and/ or trail mix;
+ baby carrots, sugar snap peas, or cherry tomatoes;
+ sliced cucumbers, celery, or green peppers;
+ fresh fruit (bags of grapes are always a big hit);
+ sliced apples with peanut butter;
+ small containers of yogurt or yogurt "squeezes";
+ small cups of organic pudding;
+ small containers of naturally sweetened applesauce— it even comes squeezable;
+ individually wrapped string cheese or other cheeses;
+ fruit leather (100 percent fruit variety from the natural food store);
+ a box of sweetened soy or rice milk, a 100 percent fruit juice box, or a bottle of pure water;

- and, of course, a yummy, low-fat, naturally sweetened cookie, cake, brownie, energy bar, or some other treat that you bought at the natural food store or made yourself (refined sugar will *not* increase your child's effectiveness for the rest of the day).

Dinner — Lighter Is Better

There is a new movement afoot in the West advocated by Dr. John Douillard, author of *The 3-Season Diet*. The movement? Eat your largest meal at lunch and supplement it with a light dinner. For you trivia buffs, that's where the word *supper* comes from — it's "supplemental." Our North American ancestors, as well as people in many countries throughout the world, not to mention prehistoric peoples, followed this routine knowing that, as the day wears on, and especially after the sun sets, the metabolism slows down, and digestive ability becomes increasingly weak. Your digestive ability is the highest when the sun is at the highest point in the sky. So, if you're going to have dinner, have it earlier (before six o'clock is best) and try some of these on-the-lighter-side recipes — and no cookies and milk before bed!

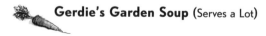 **Gerdie's Garden Soup** (Serves a Lot)

This is an excellent "kitchen sink" vegetable soup. The root vegetables give the broth a full flavor that is perfect for autumn weather.

Ingredients

2 qt filtered water

1/2 cup dried lentils (rinsed)

1/4 cup barley

Bay leaves

1 medium rutabaga

2 large yams

2 onions

3 carrots (scrub but don't peel!)

1 small head cabbage, chopped

1 can diced tomatoes

1 1/2 tbsp salt

1/2 tbsp garlic powder

1/2 tbsp ground cumin

3 stalks celery, thinly sliced

1/2 tbsp black pepper

Directions

1. Boil water in a large stock pot. Add lentils, barley, and bay leaves and let the mixture continue to boil.
2. Meanwhile, chop rutabaga, yams, onions, carrots, and cabbage until the pieces are no larger than a nickel. Add to the boiling water.
3. Add the rest of the ingredients, except celery and black pepper. Add water to fill the pot if necessary. Let boil for 10 minutes.
4. Reduce heat and simmer for 20 more minutes (or until lentils are cooked). Add celery and pepper and cook for five more minutes.

TIP: This soup is filling yet light and tasty. Parsnips or turnips are easily substituted for rutabagas when in season and add a great flavor to the soup. This soup freezes well, so feel free to cook large quantities and save a few quarts in the freezer.

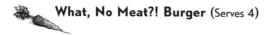

What, No Meat?! Burger (Serves 4)

This veggie burger is a personal triumph! After putting up with one too many soggy buns, I thought it was hopeless to try creating a veggie burger with the taste and texture of the real thing. Time after time, I bit into what tasted like a sloppy rice patty. I can happily say that these tasty burgers actually have the look and feel of meat burgers, and they are packed with protein from the lentils and tofu. The best part? These patties won't fall apart when cooking.

Ingredients
1 cup dry lentils
1 onion
3 cloves garlic
1 tsp chili powder
2 pkg extra firm tofu
1/3 cup whole-wheat flour
2 tbsp Pickapeppa sauce
2 tbsp Worcestershire sauce
1/2 cup real tomato ketchup
1/2 cup bread crumbs
Salt and pepper

Directions

1. Wash and rinse lentils. Place them in a saucepan and add three cups of cold water. Finely chop onion and add to lentils. Add garlic and chili powder and bring the mixture to a boil.

2. Reduce heat, cover, and simmer until lentils are tender, about 45 minutes.

3. While lentils are cooking, place tofu and whole-wheat flour in a food processor. Add Pickapeppa sauce, Worcestershire sauce, and ketchup. Blend until mixture is smooth.

4. When lentils are tender, drain thoroughly, reserving liquid. Add lentils to tofu-flour mixture and blend for one or two minutes. Add bread crumbs and mix by hand until well incorporated. Season mixture with salt and pepper.

5. The mixture should be thick and easy to spoon onto a hot griddle in the shape of burgers. Spray the griddle with non-stick spray and cook patties on each side until golden brown.

 TIP: Serve on whole-wheat buns with ketchup, pickles, lettuce, tomatoes, and onion slices—all the trimmings! You can even melt a slice of cheese or soy cheese in the last few minutes of browning. And why not cook up some French or American fries just like Mom used to make?

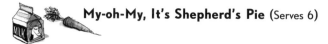

My-oh-My, It's Shepherd's Pie (Serves 6)

Traditional shepherd's pie is a hearty one-dish meal made of mashed potatoes, corn, and ground beef. This variation on an old favorite replaces the meat with beans. You can also experiment with adding soy protein to this recipe.

Ingredients
3 small potatoes
2 cloves garlic, minced
1/2 tsp dried basil
2 tbsp olive oil
1/4 tsp salt
2–4 tbsp soy milk
1 medium onion, chopped
1 medium carrot, sliced
1 tbsp olive oil
1 can kidney beans, drained
1 can whole tomatoes, drained and cut
1 cup peas
1 8 oz can tomato sauce
1 tsp Worcestershire sauce (see note)
1 tbsp sugar
1 cup grated cheddar cheese or soy cheese
Paprika

Directions

1. Peel and quarter potatoes. Cook, covered, in boiling, salted water for 20–25 minutes or until tender. Drain. Mash until smooth.

2. In a small saucepan, cook garlic and dried basil in olive oil just until golden. Add to mashed potatoes along with salt. Gradually beat in enough milk to make light and fluffy. Set aside.

3. For filling, in a medium saucepan, cook onion and carrot in hot oil until onion is tender but not brown. Stir in kidney beans, tomatoes, vegetables, tomato sauce, Worcestershire sauce, and sugar. Heat until bubbly.

4. Transfer vegetable mixture to a baking pan. Drop mashed potatoes in four mounds over vegetable mixture. Sprinkle with cheddar cheese and paprika.

5. Bake, uncovered, at 375 degrees for 25–30 minutes or until heated through and cheese begins to brown.

 Note: Regular Worcestershire sauce is not vegetarian because it contains anchovies. However, vegetarian Worcestershire sauce is available. If you are unable to find it, simply leave it out of the recipe.

Tofu Cheese Seashells (Makes 12)

The added nutrition of tofu, carrots, and spinach makes this Italian favorite an everyday vegan masterpiece.

Ingredients
12 jumbo pasta shells
1/4 cup finely grated carrot
1 green onion, sliced
1 cup chopped spinach
1 pkg firm tofu, drained
1/2 cup grated soy cheese
1 egg white or egg substitute
1/4 tsp salt
1/4 tsp pepper
Sauce
Soy Parmesan cheese

Directions
1. Cook pasta shells according to package directions. Rinse with cold water, drain, and set aside.
2. In a small saucepan, cook carrot, green onion, and spinach in a small amount of water till tender. Drain well, drying excess moisture with paper towels.
3. In a medium mixing bowl, mash drained tofu with a fork. Stir in carrot-green onion-spinach mixture, soy cheese, egg white, salt, and pepper.

4. Stuff each cooked pasta shell with one tablespoon of the filling. Place shells in an ungreased, two-quart, square baking dish. Pour your favorite sauce over shells. Cover and bake at 350 degrees for about 25 minutes or until heated through. Sprinkle with soy Parmesan cheese.

Sloppy Veggie Josies (Serves 8)

I know, I know, not exactly an adventurous recipe. However, even the vegetarian epicure will adore this recipe, well balanced in protein and carbohydrates. These sloppy Josies taste the best with kidney beans, black beans, or a combination of them, but pintos can be used for a southwestern flair. The addition of ground soy meat available in your health food grocer's freezer adds the expected texture. Don't forget to allow time to soak the beans the night before — but if you do forget, just open a can.

Ingredients
1 lb any variety of beans
1 small onion, diced
1 cup soy meat
Olive oil
3 tbsp chili powder
2 tbsp brown sugar
1 8 oz can tomato sauce
1 bag buns

Directions

1. Soak a pound of beans overnight. Rinse well and change the water. Bring to a boil. After 45 minutes, pour off excess water and continue cooking for 15 minutes.
2. Meanwhile, sauté onion and soy meat in oil. Add onion and soy meat mixture to beans and cook at medium boil.
3. Mix chili powder and sugar with a little water and add to beans. Mix in can of tomato sauce and stir well.
4. Load up the buns and enjoy.

 TIP: You can use molasses instead of brown sugar to make the mixture more cohesive. Also consider adding nuts or barley for texture.

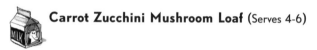 **Carrot Zucchini Mushroom Loaf** (Serves 4-6)

Here's a meat-free loaf that will amaze your nonvegetarian friends! You can make the recipe using all carrots, all zucchini, or a combination.

Ingredients

4 cloves garlic, minced
1 lb mushrooms, chopped
1 large onion, chopped
1/4 cup and 2 tbsp butter
1 cup bread crumbs, divided
1 cup grated cheese, divided

5 eggs

2 cups grated carrots

2 cups grated zucchini

2 tsp basil

1 tsp pepper

1/2 tsp salt

1/2 tsp tarragon

Directions

1. Preheat oven to 350 degrees.

2. Sauté garlic, mushrooms, and onion in a quarter cup butter until soft.

3. Combine half a cup bread crumbs and half a cup grated cheese and mix with all other ingredients, including mushrooms and onions, but reserve the 2 tbsp butter.

4. Press into a buttered loaf pan and sprinkle remaining bread crumbs and cheese over the top.

5. Dot remaining butter on the top, cover with foil, and bake for about 30 minutes. Remove foil and bake an additional five minutes or until golden brown.

 TIP: Use Swiss cheese if you're going heavy on the carrots and Cheddar if you're using more zucchini.

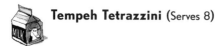 **Tempeh Tetrazzini** (Serves 8)

Ingredients

2 tbsp vegetable oil

1 shallot, chopped

1 garlic clove, minced

1 lb mushrooms, sliced

3 tbsp chopped parsley

2 tbsp thyme leaves

2 bay leaves

Salt and pepper to taste

Grated zest of one lemon

2 cups vegetable broth, low sodium

4 tbsp butter

1/4 cup flour

1 egg yolk, lightly beaten

1 cup milk or soy milk

4 lb cooked tempeh tenders

1 lb egg noodles, cooked

1/2 cup bread crumbs

1/2 cup grated Parmesan

1/2 cup sliced almonds, toasted

Directions

1. Coat a skillet with oil and put over medium heat. Add shallot and garlic. Cook, stirring, until translucent, about three minutes. Add the mushrooms and herbs and sauté for three to five minutes until lightly browned. Season with salt and pepper. Transfer the mushrooms to a glass

bowl, grate in the zest of a lemon, then cover with plastic wrap to infuse the flavor. Set aside.

2. Heat vegetable broth in a medium saucepan and keep warm over low heat. Melt butter in the skillet and stir in flour to make a roux. Cook, stirring constantly, for three minutes. Whisk in warm broth and stir vigorously to avoid lumps. Continue for five minutes until sauce is thickened and smooth. Add egg, milk, reserved mushrooms, and tempeh. Cook and stir until heated through —do not let boil. Fold in cooked noodles and mix to combine.

3. Spoon the mixture into a buttered 9- by 13-inch baking pan and smooth out with a spoon. Sprinkle with bread crumbs and Parmesan cheese. Bake at 350 degrees until the sauce bubbles and a top crust has formed, 20–30 minutes. Garnish with toasted almonds before serving.

Jammin' Jambalaya (Serves 6)

You can also get creative when it comes to some old favorites, such as jambalaya. This is one of the best examples of an old recipe with a vegetarian twist. It retains the flavors and textures of the original, due in large part to the teaspoon of liquid smoke and the tofu's chewy texture. Allow time to completely freeze and then thaw the tofu before you start to cook this dish since freezing completely changes the texture of tofu, making it chewy.

Ingredients

1 lb extra firm tofu, frozen and thawed

2 tbsp oil

1 large onion, chopped

4–6 garlic cloves, minced

1 can tomatoes, chopped, reserve liquid

1 cup water or vegetable stock

1 cup chopped celery

1 cup green bell pepper, diced

1 cup red bell pepper, diced

1 tsp liquid smoke

3/4 cup fresh parsley, minced

2 bay leaves

2 tsp dried thyme leaves

2 tsp dried basil

1/4 tsp cayenne

2 cups uncooked rice

Salt and pepper

Hot sauce (Tabasco) to taste

Directions

1. Squeeze as much water out of thawed tofu as possible, without breaking it up too much. Cut squeezed tofu into half-inch squares and set aside.

2. Heat oil in a large Dutch oven and add onions and garlic. Sauté until just starting to brown. Add all remaining ingredients except tofu, rice, and reserved liquid.

3. Combine reserved tomato juice and water or vegetable stock to make about three cups. Add this mixture to the pot and bring to a boil.
4. Add drained tofu and rice. Cover, reduce heat, and simmer for about 45 minutes.
5. Remove from heat. Remove bay leaves, and season to taste.

Snacks

Nutritionists report that a common problem with the eating habits of children is that they go too long without healthy food between meals. If you can get your children to come right home after school instead of stopping with their friends at the local convenience store, you have a fighting chance of getting something nutritious into them instead of the sugary items that might give them a burst of energy but eventually leave their blood sugar levels lower than they were before—not an ideal situation for the mental clarity they need to do their homework or the physical strength they need for sports practices or games.

By stocking your cupboards and fridge with healthy snack choices, you will encourage your vegetarian child to eat the right kinds of foods to maintain energy until dinner. Remember, you won't have to force, coax, bribe, or nag your child to eat good food if you offer appealing choices. To accomplish this, you just have to get creative with the snack foods in your kitchen. Below are a few suggestions.

Never-Empty Veggie Platter

A great "grazing" treat to always keep in the fridge is a big veggie platter with carrots, celery, sugar snap peas, broccoli, radishes, lightly steamed green beans, and a healthy dip such as hummus or even low-fat ranch dressing. Adolescents will devour this platter if it's there. And if you don't have time to cut up the veggies, most grocery stores sell precut platters. A fun variation especially for the younger kids is to fill the celery with cream cheese or peanut butter and put some raisins on the top.

Kids' Kabobs

Try mini fruit-and-cheese kabobs. They are quick and easy. Using small skewers (you can get sticks six to eight inches at almost any grocery store), thread on fruit and cheese of your choice. Kids love pineapple, strawberries, melon, and chunks of mozzarella—or try grapes, Cheddar, and apples. The choices are endless, and you can cater to your child's taste. Stack up the skewers with other delights such as veggies, tofu, even olives. You can also use pretzel sticks as skewers.

Tortilla Mania

Great snacks start with inexpensive tortillas—and these days you can even get them in whole wheat and flavored varieties such as spinach and tomato. Children like grated cheese melted on a tortilla folded and cut into wedges. To pack them with more vitamins and fiber, add finely grated veggies and/or some refried or whole beans. Serve salsa on the side for a health-ful dip. (Did you know that the US government considers salsa a vegetable?) You can also try tortilla roll-ups by spreading cream cheese and thinly sliced veggies on the tortillas and then rolling and slicing them up.

Dried Fruit and Nuts

A delicious and healthy snack to always have on hand is your own homemade trail mix. Use your creativity and mix soy nuts with raisins, chopped dates, or any favorite dried fruit. Try dried apricots, dried cranberries, walnut pieces, sunflower seeds, or almonds. You can always throw in a few chocolate or carob chips for a special treat. In Debra's house, they have a covered acrylic candy dish in the kitchen with raisins in one section, pis-tachios in one, and trail mix in the other two. This is a great snack for the entire family—and the kids don't even miss the M&M's.

Deviled Eggs

If your kids aren't vegans, they probably love hard-boiled eggs. If you have them in your fridge, they'll probably be happy to grab one and peel it. But just to make it even easier and tastier for them to partake in this nutritious snack, boil the eggs, let them cool, cut them in half, remove the yolk, mix it with a bit of mayo, salt, and pepper, and put the mixture back into the egg halves. You'll be surprised at how fast they disappear! To reduce fat content, replace the yolks with tofu.

Peanut Butter Passion

Peanut butter is an excellent source of protein for vegetarians. And it's easy for moms who want to whip up quick, tasty snacks. True, peanut butter is high in fat. But most of it is mono-unsaturated, the same "good fat" found in olive oil. Yes, it's also high in calories, so here are some ways to use peanut butter sparingly.

Use it as a flavorful spread on fruit such as apples and pears or on frozen bananas. Try it on graham crackers, bread, and bagels. Some even like peanut butter on their pretzels. For a special treat, give in to the perennial kids' favorite of peanut butter balls. Although high in fat, they also provide a lot of high-quality protein, iron, and vitamins. Just combine a cup of peanut butter with sweetened coconut, non-fat dry milk, raisins, and honey. Mix together, form into balls, and eat. They should be refrigerated.

Mini Pizzas

Using half a bagel or English muffin, create kid-size pizzas. Spoon on some pizza sauce and top with whatever vegetables suit your fancy. Any toppings will do. I like spinach topped with a few tomato slices and then sprinkled with soy or Parmesan cheese. If you wish, pop the pizzas under the broiler for a minute or so to brown the cheese. Warm through, cut into slices, and eat. Other great veggies to add include green peppers, mushrooms, even zucchini. Some love the taste of pineapple on pizza. You can also substitute any leftover cooked or frozen veggies you have on hand.

Frozen Snacks

There's always healthful and delicious frozen yogurt, but if your child is vegan there are many frozen confections at the natural food store made from rice and soy. Kids particularly love frozen fruit juice bars, which you can easily make, and they love the chunks of fruit (especially watermelon) in the store-bought brand, and they love frozen bananas.

And Then There's Always . . . Good Old Fresh Fruit

If you cut it, they will eat it.

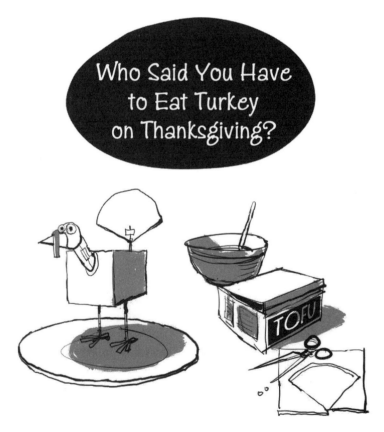

CHAPTER 5

Who Said You Have to Eat Turkey on Thanksgiving?

Emily's Vegetarian Cooking for Special Occasions

By now, you've probably become quite the expert at vegetarian meal preparation. You have the day-to-day meals down, and you've even tried out some of the more adventurous recipes on your family. You're getting used to the idea that your child is committed to this new lifestyle — but, wait, now we're talking Thanksgiving dinner! There is no way you are going to serve your child a tofu turkey! He can make an exception at least one day of the year so he doesn't completely ruin your family holiday.

Calm down. I understand how you feel. A large part of holiday celebrations centers on food. The "family meal" is not only about delicious once-a-year delicacies but about the customs and traditions passed across the generations such as Aunt Flo's Famous Thanksgiving Turkey, Grandma Betty's World-Renowned Easter Ham, or Bubbe's Special Passover Roast Beef. With each holiday, the family meal is the focal point of the day and is often planned and prepared for way in advance. How are you supposed to feel when your vegetarian child doesn't want to participate in these cherished family traditions?

Let's consider traditions for what they *truly* are. They give form and expression to our holiday celebrations. They give us ways of relating to each other and creating memories. Traditions aren't necessarily the right way to do things; they are simply what your family has done since before you were even born. It's not the physical food that makes the holiday but the love and togetherness the food creates. Love is the true gift of the season, and to allow your child's food choices to harm that love would be unfortunate.

Why not look at this year as an opportunity to start a new tradition by adding a vegetarian dish to your standard holiday feast? Acceptance and compromise will add to the holiday spirit. Rejection and rigidity will only diminish it.

This chapter offers vegetarian and vegan holiday recipes that will complement traditional menus or stand on their own. By preparing a few of these dishes, you can show your vegetarian child that nothing is more important than the *people* at the dinner table.

Thanksgiving

Did you know that there is no evidence that turkey was served at the Pilgrims' first Thanksgiving? Why, then, has it become such an indispensable part of the Thanksgiving tradition?

Thanksgiving turkey is rooted in the *History of Plymouth Plantation*, written by William Bradford some 22 years after the actual celebration. In this letter sent to another Pilgrim,

Bradford described how the governor sent "four men out fowling," and they returned with turkeys, ducks, and geese. The Bradford letter was lost during the War of Independence and wasn't rediscovered until 1854. Since then, turkey has been a popular symbol of America's Thanksgiving Day.

History aside, for many, a turkey dinner is incomplete without its vegetarian counterparts: mashed potatoes, sweet potatoes, green beans, and cranberry sauce. Thanksgiving should present no problem for your vegetarian child even without any special preparation. But just in case you want to do a bit extra, this section offers popular recipes for vegetarians and vegans that all the guests at your dining room table can enjoy.

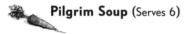 **Pilgrim Soup** (Serves 6)

This flavorful recipe is a great start for Thanksgiving dinner. The warm colors and fragrant aroma will tantalize the taste buds in preparation for the meal to come.

Ingredients
1 large butternut squash, peeled, seeded, and cubed
1 small onion, cut in wedges
1 Granny Smith apple, peeled, cored, and cubed
4 cups water
1 tbsp sugar
2 tsp vegetable broth powder
1/2 tsp crushed rosemary
1 cup soy milk

Directions

1. Combine the squash, onion, apple, water, sugar, vegetable broth powder, and rosemary in a soup pot. Bring to a boil, reduce heat, and simmer until the squash is very tender, 30–40 minutes.
2. Purée soup in a blender until smooth. You may want to let it cool a little first. Return soup to the pot.
3. Stir the soy milk into the soup and heat gently until warm.

 TIP: Serve topped with seasoned croutons.

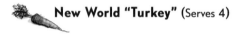 **New World "Turkey"** (Serves 4)

This is a simple vegan alternative to turkey. Try it out on meat eaters, and they may well ask for seconds! Don't worry; it is much less time consuming than it appears.

Ingredients
1 lb firm tofu
1 tsp salt
1/4 tsp dried marjoram
1/4 tsp dried savory
1/4 tsp pepper
1 pkg dry bread stuffing mix
2/3 cup water
1/4 cup soy margarine

1 slice bread, cubed

1/2 tsp sage

2 tbsp water

5 tbsp vegetable oil, divided

1 tsp barbecue sauce

1/2 tsp mustard

1 tbsp orange jam

1 tsp orange juice

1 tbsp sesame seeds

Directions

1. Drain and rinse tofu; in a food processor or blender, process tofu until smooth. Stir in salt, marjoram, savory, and pepper.
2. Line a sieve with two sheets of paper towel and place over an empty bowl. Place tofu in lined sieve and press against sides to form a deep well in the middle. Place two more sheets of paper towel over tofu and refrigerate for two hours.
3. Meanwhile, in a medium saucepan over medium-high heat, combine stuffing mix, two-thirds cup water, and margarine. Bring to a boil; reduce heat to low, cover, and simmer for five minutes. Remove from heat; let stand five minutes and fluff with a fork. To this mixture add bread cubes, sage, and two tablespoons water.
4. After tofu has chilled for two hours, preheat oven to 350 degrees. With two tablespoons of vegetable oil, grease a baking sheet.

5. Remove top layer of paper towels from tofu. If necessary, again press tofu against sides of the sieve to form a well. Spoon stuffing mixture into the well and smooth surface with a spoon. Invert tofu mold onto prepared baking sheet. Remove remaining paper towel layer and shape tofu with your hands if it has cracked or lost its shape.

6. Bake in preheated oven for 30 minutes.

7. Meanwhile, prepare glaze by combining barbecue sauce, mustard, orange jam, orange juice, sesame seeds, and remaining three tablespoons of oil.

8. After tofu has baked for 30 minutes, brush glaze over it. Return it to the oven and bake for 20 minutes more. At the end, broil for three to five minutes or until tofu is browned and crispy. Serve with vegan gravy (below).

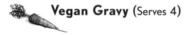 **Vegan Gravy** (Serves 4)

This light and flavorful gravy is the perfect accompaniment to New World "Turkey."

Ingredients
2 cans vegetable broth
2 cloves garlic, pressed
1/2 small onion, thinly sliced
1/2 cup mushrooms, thinly sliced
1/2 tsp salt
1/2 tsp pepper
1/2 tsp savory

1/2 tsp thyme

1 tsp rosemary

Parsley, to taste

1/3 cup water

2 tbsp cornstarch

Directions

1. Pour vegetable broth into a pan. Add garlic, onion, mushrooms, and spices. Bring to a boil; then reduce heat and let simmer for 30 minutes or more. The longer you let it simmer, the more flavorful it will be.

2. In a bowl with one-third cup water, add one tablespoon of cornstarch and mix until smooth. Add to vegetable broth. Bring to a boil while stirring often. Thicken to your liking by adding more cornstarch.

Alicia's Cranberry Sauce

This cranberry sauce gets rave reviews. Celery and walnuts add unexpected flavor and crunch. Have a few copies of the recipe handy—your friends and family will request this one for sure!

Ingredients

1 pkg cherry flavor gelatin (see tip below)

2 cups boiling water

1/2 cup ice cubes

1 can whole cranberry sauce

1 can crushed pineapple, undrained

1/2 cup chopped walnuts

1/2 cup finely chopped celery

Directions

1. Pour gelatin into boiling water. Stir for two to three minutes or until all powder is dissolved.
2. Add half a cup of ice cubes and stir until they have melted.
3. Add all other ingredients.
4. Stir well and pour into mold. Refrigerate until set, usually about six hours.

 TIP: Gelatin is made from animal by-products, but Hain's offers a vegetarian variety that may be purchased at your local natural food store. So you can still make Jell-O molds and salads!

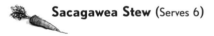 **Sacagawea Stew** (Serves 6)

This stew is packed with vitamins and protein from squash, corn, and beans. These vegetables are perfect for the harvest festival of Thanksgiving.

Ingredients

1 large butternut squash

1 tbsp olive oil

1 medium onion, chopped

2 cloves garlic, minced

1/2 medium green pepper, cut into short, narrow strips

1 16 oz can diced tomatoes, with liquid

2 cups cooked or canned pinto beans

2 cups corn kernels

1 cup vegetable stock or water

1 small fresh hot chili, seeded and minced

1 tsp ground cumin

1 tsp dried oregano

Salt and freshly ground black pepper

3–4 tbsp minced fresh cilantro

Directions

1. Preheat oven to 400 degrees.
2. Cut squash in half lengthwise and remove seeds and fibers. Place halves, cut side up, in a shallow baking pan and cover with aluminum foil. Bake for 45 minutes or until easily pierced with a knife but still firm. When cool enough to handle, scoop out pulp and cut into large cubes. Set aside.
3. Heat oil in a soup pot. Add onion and sauté over medium-low heat until translucent. Add garlic and continue to sauté until onion is golden. Add squash and all remaining ingredients except cilantro and bring to a simmer.
4. Simmer gently, covered, until vegetables are tender, about 20 to 25 minutes. Season to taste with salt and pepper. Just before serving, stir in cilantro.

TIP: The stew should be thick and moist but not soupy; add additional stock or water if needed.

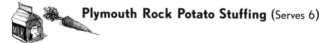 **Plymouth Rock Potato Stuffing** (Serves 6)

This hearty stuffing is a fulfilling and delicious side dish.

Ingredients

6 potatoes, cooked in their skins
1 cup low-fat milk or soy milk
4 slices whole-grain bread
1 1/2 tbsp light olive oil
1 cup chopped onion
1 cup chopped celery
1/4 cup finely chopped fresh parsley
2 tsp herb and spice mixture of your choice
Salt and freshly ground black pepper

Directions

1. Preheat oven to 350 degrees.
2. Once cooked potatoes are cool enough to handle, peel and place them in a large mixing bowl. Coarsely mash potatoes with half a cup of milk or unsweetened soy milk.
3. Cut bread into half-inch cubes. Put them into a small mixing bowl and pour remaining milk or soy milk over them. Soak for several minutes.
4. Meanwhile, heat oil in a medium-sized skillet. Add onion and celery and sauté over low heat until onion is lightly browned and celery is tender.

5. Combine onion and celery mixture with mashed potatoes in the large mixing bowl. Stir in soaked bread,
parsley, spices, and mix well. Season to taste with salt
and pepper. Pour mixture into a well-oiled, two-quart
baking dish. Bake for 55 minutes or until top is a crusty
golden brown.

Grandma Beverly's Sweet Potatoes (Serves 10)

Sweet potatoes don't need miniature marshmallows for delec-
table sweetness. This recipe uses dried apricots instead. This
was one of Debra's mother-in-law's favorites, and she was into
healthy vegetarian cooking way before the rest of us.

Ingredients
3/4 lb dried apricots
1 can apricot nectar
3/4 cup water
3 lb sweet potatoes
3/8 cup light brown sugar
4 tbsp melted butter
1 1/2 tbsp orange juice
1 tbsp orange zest
1/2 cup pecan halves

Directions

1. Place apricots in a medium saucepan and cover with apricot nectar and water. Let stand one hour. Then place over medium heat and simmer uncovered until apricots are tender (45 minutes). Cool and drain, reserving liquid.

2. Place sweet potatoes on a baking sheet and bake at 425 degrees until tender when pierced with a fork (35 minutes). Cool, peel, and cut into lengthwise slices approximately a quarter-inch thick.

3. Lightly grease a 9- by 11-inch baking dish. Arrange a layer of potatoes, then apricots, then potatoes, then apricots, and then sprinkle with brown sugar.

4. In a small bowl, mix half of the reserved liquid with melted butter, orange juice, and orange zest. Pour over potato mixture and bake uncovered at 375 degrees for 40 minutes, basting occasionally.

5. Remove from oven and place pecan halves on top. Return to oven and bake another five to 10 minutes. Let stand 10 minutes before serving.

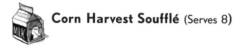 **Corn Harvest Soufflé** (Serves 8)

Some people like corn bread; others like corn as a side dish. Nothing combines the best of both like this light and fluffy soufflé.

Ingredients

2 cans whole-kernel corn

2 cans creamed corn

4 tbsp white sugar

4 tbsp all-purpose flour

4 tbsp milk or soy milk

4 eggs

Directions

1. Preheat oven to 350 degrees.
2. Combine all ingredients. Mix well. Pour mixture into a soufflé bowl.
3. Bake at 350 degrees for one to one and a half hours, until top is brown.

Vegan Pumpkin Patch Pie (Serves 8)

Pumpkin pie is a must on Thanksgiving Day. This recipe is a hands-down winner. No one needs to know that it's nondairy!

Ingredients

1 can puréed pumpkin

3/4 cup sugar

1/2 tsp salt

1 tsp ground cinnamon

1/2 tsp ground ginger

1/4 tsp ground cloves

1 pkg (10–12 oz) soft tofu, processed in blender until smooth

1 9-inch unbaked pie shell (or your own homemade pie crust)

Directions

1. Preheat oven to 425 degrees. Cream pumpkin and sugar. Add salt, spices, and tofu, mixing thoroughly. Pour mixture into pie shell and bake for 15 minutes.
2. Lower heat to 350 degrees and bake for another 40 minutes. Chill and serve.

TIP: This pie is delicious with nondairy topping or whipped cream for lacto-ovos. Don't use the low-fat tofu—the pie will taste like it was made with tofu.

Christmas

Some of the most evocative memories of Christmas are the smells and tastes of food. The extravagance of the Christmas meal was established in the Middle Ages, when feudal lords hosted meals for their serfs. Despite the long history of the Christmas feast, no universal "traditional" meal has emerged. Unlike Thanksgiving, which centers on "the bird," Christmas boasts a variety of meal traditions ranging from roast beef and turkey to more exotic meals such as Italian and Mexican feasts. But one thing is consistently central to Christmas Day—the big Christmas dinner.

The Christmas meal lives in our imaginations as endless mounds of food, drink, and dessert enjoyed in the glow of the Christmas tree lights. And afterward, we all have to "loosen our belts." Let's face it; few of us watch what we eat at Christmas — although a lot of us sure do afterward!

Why not take the lead from your vegetarian child and try out a few of these lower-calorie, nutritious, vegetarian delights? These recipes focus on elegant, simple dishes that can be easily prepared amid the caroling, gift hunting, hot-mulled wine, and vegan eggnog.

Jolly Vegan Eggnog (Serves 4)

Anyone with elevated cholesterol should eye the pitcher of eggnog with hesitation. This vegan alternative packs in the flavor without the saturated fat and cholesterol of traditional varieties.

Ingredients
1 pkg silken tofu
1/4 tsp turmeric
2 cups vanilla soy milk
1 tbsp vanilla extract
1/4 cup sugar
2 tbsp brown sugar
1/2–1 cup rum or brandy
Nutmeg to taste

Directions

1. In a blender or food processor, combine all ingredients except nutmeg and blend thoroughly.
2. Serve well chilled and dusted with nutmeg.

 TIP: This eggnog is very susceptible to the flavor of alcohol. You may want to start with smaller amounts and add more as necessary —it's even delicious with none at all.

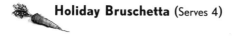 **Holiday Bruschetta** (Serves 4)

This "red and green" bruschetta looks seasonally appropriate as a premeal nibbler.

Ingredients

1 can butter beans, drained

2 cloves garlic, peeled and pressed

4 tbsp olive oil

Juice of 1/2 lemon

Roasted red and green peppers, chopped

3 tbsp tomato paste

3 tomatoes, peeled and diced

1 can black olives, chopped

Salt and pepper to taste

Ciabatta bread

Olive oil for drizzling

Directions

1. Mash butter beans roughly with garlic and add enough olive oil to make a paste.
2. Stir in lemon juice, red and green peppers, tomato paste, tomatoes, black olives, and seasonings.
3. Slice ciabatta bread and toast under the grill. Drizzle with olive oil and serve topped with butter bean mixture.

 TIP: Sprinkle with fresh grated Parmesan cheese if your teen is lacto-ovo.

Stocking Stuffed Mushrooms (Makes 8)

The beauty of this mushroom side dish is that it can be prepared a day in advance to relieve some of the kitchen madness of Christmas day. Who says mushrooms need to be deep-fried or filled with cheese to taste scrumptious?

Ingredients

8 extra-large mushrooms
1 small onion, finely chopped
1 tbsp olive oil
1/2 cup seasoned bread crumbs
1 tsp dried marjoram
1/4 cup pine nuts
1 can sweet corn
Black pepper
Pinch of salt
Fresh parsley

Directions

1. Wipe mushrooms clean. Remove and finely chop stems. Set aside.
2. Sauté half onion in olive oil. Add mushroom stems. Once tender, remove from heat.
3. Thoroughly mix in bread crumbs, marjoram, pine nuts, sweet corn, plenty of freshly ground black pepper, and pinch of salt.
4. Place mushroom caps in a shallow oven dish and pile filling into them. Dot them with a little oil.
5. Bake at 350 degrees for 20 minutes and garnish with fresh parsley. Serve hot.

North Pole Nut Roast (Serves 4-6)

Even the most obstinate meat eaters will love this healthy roast. The nutty flavor is excellent with vegan gravy.

Ingredients

1 1/2 cups finely chopped leeks
1/4 cup oil
4 tomatoes, peeled and chopped
2 cups chopped mushrooms
1 1/2 cups chopped onion
1 1/2 cups fine bread crumbs
1 cup ground almonds
1 cup ground cashews

1 cup ground hazelnuts

1 large green apple, grated

1/2 cup chopped celery

3 tbsp chopped fresh parsley

1 tsp basil

1 tsp thyme

1/2 tsp sage

1/4 tsp paprika

3 tsp egg substitute in 3 tbsp water

3 tbsp tamari

Directions

1. Gently sauté leeks in oil until soft but not browned. Put them into a large bowl. Add all remaining ingredients except for egg substitute and tamari. Mix well.

2. Add egg substitute and tamari. Stir well. Allow to stand for 10 minutes; then firmly pack into oiled five-inch by nine-inch loaf pan.

3. Place loaf pan in a baking dish and add water halfway up the loaf pan. Bake at 400 degrees for one hour, and then reduce heat to 350 degrees for another one and a half hours.

4. The top should be dark brown but not black. Allow roast to stand for five minutes before loosening sides and turning out onto serving platter.

 TIP: This is excellent the next day cold on a sandwich.

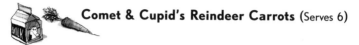 **Comet & Cupid's Reindeer Carrots** (Serves 6)

This is an excellent and aesthetic way of serving beta-carotene packed carrots!

Ingredients
1 1/2 lb carrots
8 oz baby onions
4 tbsp butter or olive oil
Juice of 1 lemon
1/2 tsp sugar
Fresh parsley, chopped

Directions
1. Preheat oven to 325 degrees.
2. Peel carrots. If you're using baby ones, leave them whole. Otherwise cut carrots into even-sized pieces.
3. Peel onions and halve or quarter any large ones.
4. Use half the butter to grease an ovenproof dish generously. Put carrots and onions into it and add lemon juice and sugar. Dot the remaining butter over surface. Cover the casserole dish and bake for about 45 minutes, until vegetables are tender.
5. Taste and add more sugar if necessary. Then sprinkle some chopped parsley over top and serve from the dish.

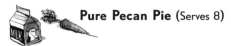

Pure Pecan Pie (Serves 8)

Ingredients

3 eggs

2/3 cup brown sugar

1/2 tsp salt

1/3 cup butter or margarine, melted

1 cup dark or light corn syrup

1 9-inch unbaked pie shell (or your own homemade
   pie crust)

1 cup pecan halves or broken pecans

Directions

1. Preheat oven to 375 degrees.
2. Beat together eggs, sugar, salt, butter, and syrup.
3. Cover bottom of pie shell with pecans.
4. Pour mixture over nuts.
5. Bake 40–50 minutes or until filling is set.

Hanukkah

There's nothing like Jewish holiday time to excite your taste buds, especially when Bubbe's around to do the cooking. Although Hanukkah is not one of the most religiously significant holidays of the Jewish calendar, its rich tradition of spinning the dreidel, lighting the eight candles (one for each night of the celebration), and watching the children reenact the story of Judah the Maccabee fosters dear memories. And, happily enough, since the holiday meal centers on potato latkes (pancakes), it is easily vegetarian! If latkes aren't enough for your family, just cook up some New World turkey with vegan gravy or some recipes from the Passover section; add kugel or blintzes, a vegetable, and a dessert, and your family will be content until the last little Maccabee is tucked into bed.

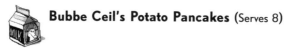 **Bubbe Ceil's Potato Pancakes** (Serves 8)

Debra says her mom is the best cook on the planet, and she really shines at holiday time. Here is her recipe for potato latkes.

Ingredients
8 large potatoes
Lemon juice
5 eggs, beaten
3/4 cup chopped onion, excess moisture squeezed off
2 tsp salt
3/4 tsp white pepper
1 1/4 tsp baking powder
1/2 cup plus 1 tbsp flour
Oil for frying

Directions

1. Wash, scrub, and grate potatoes, squeezing off all excess water. Add a few teaspoons of lemon juice to keep the white color. Add beaten eggs, onion, salt, and pepper. Then add baking powder and flour.
2. Drop rounded tablespoonfuls into hot oil and fry until deep golden brown, turning once. Remove and drain excess oil by placing on paper towels.

 TIP: Don't make them too thick, or they'll be uncooked in the middle. You can keep them warm on a baking pan in the oven until ready to eat. Serve with applesauce or sour cream. (Bubbe has relinquished her secret: use peanut oil!)

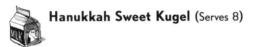 **Hanukkah Sweet Kugel** (Serves 8)

This kugel is great for any holiday or Sunday brunch.

Ingredients

8 oz pkg cream cheese

1/4 lb melted butter

1/2 cup sugar

1 tsp vanilla

Salt

2 cups milk

4 eggs

1/2 lb broad egg noodles, cooked al dente and drained

16 oz can pineapple tidbits

Maple syrup and cornflake crumbs for topping

Directions

1. Preheat oven to 350 degrees.
2. Cream together cream cheese and butter; then add sugar, vanilla, and a pinch of salt.
3. Scald milk and mix with cheese mixture. After it cools, add four eggs. Mix together. Add noodles and thoroughly drained pineapple.
4. Put in 9- by 13-inch greased baking dish and cover with thin layer of cornflake crumbs. Over that drizzle maple syrup.
5. Bake at 350 degrees for up to an hour and 15 minutes.

The Best Broccoli Casserole Ever (Serves 8)

If your kids are like most, they can't like broccoli just on the principle of the thing. But this casserole is so good that even Big Mac lovers will ask for more.

Ingredients

1 lb fresh broccoli spears
2 eggs, beaten
1 16 oz can stewed tomatoes
1 can Cheddar cheese soup
Parmesan cheese
Oregano

Directions

1. Cook (but do not overcook) broccoli. Put in buttered 9-by 13-inch casserole dish with one stem one way and the next stem the other way.
2. Pour beaten eggs over broccoli. Next pour in stewed tomatoes and finally Cheddar cheese soup. Sprinkle with Parmesan cheese (heavily) and oregano and bake at 350 degrees for 30 minutes.

Vegan "Cheese" Blintzes with Blueberry Sauce
(Makes 8)

Hanukkah desserts, such as jelly doughnuts, are traditionally deep-fried, but since this meal includes fried latkes it might be prudent to opt for a healthier version of "cheese" blintzes made with tofu.

Ingredients

Sauce 2 cups blueberries

1/3 cup light brown sugar, or to taste

Dash lemon juice

2 tbsp cornstarch

Blintz 1 1/2 cups whole-wheat pastry flour

Batter 1/2 tsp salt

3 egg substitutes, beaten

1 1/4 cups water

1 cup soy milk

2 tbsp safflower oil

Filling   1 1/2 lb soft, well-mashed tofu

3 tbsp honey, or to taste

1 tsp lemon juice

1/2 tsp cinnamon

Directions

1. Combine blueberries, sugar, and lemon juice in a food processor. Pulse until blueberries are coarsely chopped. Sprinkle in cornstarch and pulse a few more times. Transfer mixture to a saucepan and bring to a simmer. Simmer until mixture has thickened. Remove from the heat and let cool to room temperature.

2. Combine flour and salt in a mixing bowl. In another bowl, combine egg substitute with water, soy milk, and oil. Stir until well blended. Make a well in the flour and pour wet mixture into it. Stir vigorously until smoothly combined — don't overbeat.

3. Heat a 6- or 7-inch non-stick skillet. When it is hot enough to make a drop of water sizzle, drop a quarter-cup of batter in and swirl it around until it coats the skillet. Cook on both sides until golden. Remove to a plate and repeat until batter is used up.

4. Combine ingredients for the filling in a small mixing bowl. If "cheese" seems very dry, add some soy milk to give it a creamier consistency. Divide mixture among pancakes and fold. Serve at room temperature, passing the sauce around for guests to spoon over their blintzes.

Passover

For most Jewish adults, their most vivid holiday memories are those of the Passover dinner with the symbolic seder plate in the middle of the table and the cup of wine filled to the brim waiting for the prophet Elijah to come and drink. Since no leavening is allowed in any of the foods, Passover foods used to taste about as exciting as the matzo. But as Debra's mother says, "You don't have to suffer at Passover anymore." With generations of *balibustas* experimenting with ways to make the Passover feast one that tantalizes the taste buds, you'll be amazed at the delicious flavors of these foods—and they're all vegetarian!

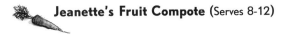 **Jeanette's Fruit Compote** (Serves 8-12)

The simplest and best compote I've ever tasted comes from Debra's neighbor Jeanette.

Ingredients
2 lb prunes
1 lb dried apricots
8 dried pears
2 handfuls white raisins
Purified water
1 slice lemon
2 sticks cinnamon
1/2 cup sugar

Directions

1. Put fruits in a saucepan. Cover with purified water and let stand overnight.
2. Add one slice lemon, two sticks cinnamon, and some more water.
3. Bring to a boil for one minute.
4. After cooled, add half a cup sugar.

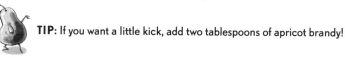 **TIP:** If you want a little kick, add two tablespoons of apricot brandy!

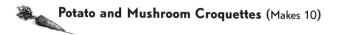 **Potato and Mushroom Croquettes** (Makes 10)

A fabulous "main course" for Passover vegetarians — and delicious as a side dish for the rest of the family.

Ingredients

1 1/2 lb potatoes, peeled and chopped

1 onion, peeled and chopped

1/4 lb mushrooms

1 tsp plus 1 tbsp oil

1 tbsp water

Salt and pepper to taste

1 cup matzo meal

Directions
1. Boil potatoes until tender. Drain and mash potatoes. In a separate pan, sauté onions and mushrooms in oil over medium-high heat for three minutes.
2. In a large bowl, mix mashed potatoes, sautéed onions and mushrooms, seasonings, and matzo meal.
3. Form 10 croquettes. Heat oil in a large frying pan over medium-high heat and fry croquettes for eight minutes on each side.

Eggplant Casserole (Serves 8)

A wonderful vegetable dish for when you can't look at another string bean—or a delicious main course for one of the other nights of Passover.

Ingredients
3 tbsp oil
1 large onion, chopped
1 medium eggplant, peeled and cubed
1/4 cup diced green pepper
1 can tomato sauce
Fresh mushrooms
1 tsp salt
1/2 tsp pepper
2 large tomatoes, diced
1 1/2 cups matzo farfel

Directions

1. Sauté onions in oil until tender. Combine onions, eggplant, green pepper, mushrooms, tomato sauce, and seasoning.
2. Cook, covered, for 15 minutes or until eggplant is tender. Stir in tomatoes. In a two-quart baking dish, arrange in alternate layers vegetables and matzo farfel. Begin and end with vegetables.
3. Bake at 350 degrees (uncovered) for 25 minutes.

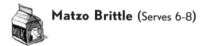 **Matzo Brittle** (Serves 6-8)

Just when you thought it was truly impossible to find a Passover dessert with fewer than 16 eggs in it, this matzo brittle shows up.

Ingredients

1/2 box matzo

2 sticks butter

1 cup brown sugar

12 oz bag chocolate chips

1 cup chopped nuts

Directions

1. Line cookie sheet with foil and cover with matzos.
2. Melt two butter sticks and mix with brown sugar until smooth. Pour over matzos.

3. Bake for five minutes at 375 degrees. Pour chocolate chips on top and spread. Sprinkle with chopped nuts. Break in pieces when cool.

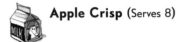

Apple Crisp (Serves 8)

Another eggless Passover wonder.

Ingredients
6 apples, peeled, cored, and sliced
1/2 cup sugar
1/2 tsp cinnamon
1/2 tsp nutmeg
2 tsp lemon juice
1/2 cup sugar
1/4 cup matzo cake meal
1/8 tsp salt
6 tbsp butter
1/4 cup chopped nuts

Directions
1. In a bowl, combine apples, first half-cup sugar, cinnamon, nutmeg, and lemon juice.
2. Pour into greased 1 1/2-quart casserole dish.

3. In a bowl, blend to crumbly consistency next half-cup sugar, matzo cake meal, salt, and butter.
   Sprinkle mixture over apples. Bake at 350 degrees for one hour until crust is nicely browned.
4. Top with chopped nuts.

Two More Jewish Holiday Treats

Chopped "Liver" Spread (Serves 8-12)

What's a holiday without a little chopped liver?

Ingredients
5 tbsp oil
1 lb mushrooms, chopped
1 medium onion, chopped
1 3/4 cups chopped walnuts
Pepper and salt, to taste
2 tbsp water (or as needed)

Directions
1. Heat oil and sauté mushrooms and onion for eight minutes. Pour into a blender or food processor, adding walnuts, seasonings, and water.
2. Blend until smooth. Serve on matzo as a spread.

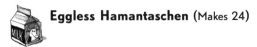 **Eggless Hamantaschen** (Makes 24)

I doubted that I would find an eggless recipe for hamantaschen, but Debra's friend Lisa came through! I found these easier to make and more delicious than my old recipe.

Ingredients
2 cups flour
2 sticks margarine or butter (room temperature)
2 tbsp sugar
8 oz cream cheese (room temperature)
1 1/2 cup jam or jelly

Directions
1. Mix flour, margarine, sugar, and cream cheese together with hands. Knead until doughy consistency forms and form into a large ball.
2. Divide into 24 little balls and refrigerate overnight.
3. Pat balls flat, put one tablespoon of jam or jelly in the center of each, and pinch up on three sides. Bake at 350 degrees for 25 minutes or until golden brown.

Easter

In many families, honey-glazed hams are to Easter what turkeys are to Thanksgiving: a once-a-year holiday tradition. The customary Easter ham is believed to have its roots in the cold countries of northern and central Europe. In Hungary and neighboring countries, the last hams and pork roasts of winter storage are served as a celebration of spring's new bounty. Southern Europeans in Mediterranean countries, where lambs are far more plentiful than pigs, serve lamb instead. For Europeans observing Lent, a feast of ham or lamb is a grand meal, especially following weeks of dining without meat.

There aren't many tofu recipes that mimic the flavor and texture of the Easter ham. However, there are some pretty good "soy hams" in the cold-cuts aisle of your natural food store. But even without the ham, there are many traditional Easter menu items for vegetarians that I'm sure every bunny will love.

April Apple Salad (Serves 8)

This light and healthy start to Easter dinner ruins the reputation of salads as green! The sweetness of the apples complements the flavors of any Easter menu.

Ingredients
1/2 cup Nayonnaise
1/2 cup applesauce
1–2 tbsp honey

1 tbsp fresh lemon juice

1/4 tsp salt

3 large Golden Delicious apples

3 stalks celery hearts, chopped

1/2 cup sunflower seeds or walnuts

1/2 cup golden seedless raisins

Directions

1. In a large bowl, whisk together soy mayo, applesauce, honey, lemon juice, and salt; set aside.
2. Peel, core, and dice apples. Toss lightly with dressing. Add celery, seeds, and raisins. If you've got a raisin lover in the family, feel free to add more. Chill and serve.

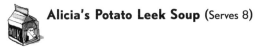 **Alicia's Potato Leek Soup** (Serves 8)

This recipe is passed down from my mother. Don't let the simplicity fool you—it tastes like a gourmet soup!

Ingredients

4 tbsp butter

8 leeks

8 cups water

6 potatoes, peeled and diced

Salt and pepper

Chervil or parsley

Directions

1. Melt butter in a large soup pot. Wash leeks thoroughly, cut into small round slices, and add to butter. Sauté leeks for two to three minutes; then add water and potatoes. Cook soup over medium heat for about an hour.

2. When soup is done, add salt and pepper according to taste, mash potatoes a bit inside soup, and stir well. As you serve each bowl, sprinkle a bit of well-minced chervil, or parsley if you prefer, on top.

 TIP: If you want to enrich the flavor, use veggie-chicken broth instead of water. This soup is delicious served in a bread bowl with cheese (try dill havarti) and croutons.

Vegan Scalloped Potatoes (Serves 6)

Potatoes have a magical ability to convey mom, family dinner, and all the other triggers of comfort food. But mashed isn't the only variety to consider for your Easter meal. These low-fat vegan scalloped potatoes are superb.

Ingredients

4 medium potatoes

1 1/2 cups soy milk

2 tbsp flour

1 tsp salt (or seasoned salt)

1/2 – 1 tsp garlic powder

1/2 tsp paprika

1 medium onion, chopped

Dash of nutmeg

Directions

1. Peel and slice potatoes thinly. In a saucepan, combine soy milk, flour, salt, garlic powder, and paprika and cook over medium heat until sauce thickens. Add onion.
2. Layer casserole dish with half of potato slices. Spoon half of sauce over slices and repeat with remaining potatoes and sauce. Top should be covered in sauce so the potatoes don't get too brown.
3. Cover and bake in preheated oven at 350 degrees for 65 minutes.

 TIP: Feel free to use real garlic instead of powder, and add some herbs of choice such as rosemary or sage.

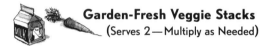 **Garden-Fresh Veggie Stacks**
(Serves 2—Multiply as Needed)

This vegetarian entrée is guaranteed to impress kids and adults. This is one recipe that looks as good as it tastes!

Ingredients

Marinade 1 tbsp garlic, chopped or pressed

1/3 cup balsamic vinegar

1/3 cup olive oil

1 tbsp basil

Stacks   4 slices eggplant, 1/3 inch each
1 yellow squash, in 1/3 inch slices
2 slices red onion, 1/3 inch each
2 large Portobello mushrooms
4 thick slices tomato
2 tbsp grated Parmesan cheese (or soy cheese)
4 slices cheese (or soy cheese)
2 stalks fresh rosemary

Directions

1. Combine all marinade ingredients in a small bowl. In a separate large bowl, combine eggplant, squash, and red onion. Pour marinade over these vegetables and let sit for half an hour. Add mushrooms and toss lightly; then let sit for five minutes.
2. Preheat oven to 450 degrees. Brush a baking sheet with oil. Remove vegetables from marinade and arrange in a single layer on the baking sheet. Roast for 10 to 15 minutes or until browned and tender. Add sliced tomatoes at the end since they need to roast for only three to five minutes. Keep a close watch on them, or they will completely fall apart. Remove vegetables from oven.
3. Oil a new baking dish. Place Portobello mushrooms on the sheet. Sprinkle Parmesan over mushrooms. Top with one slice of eggplant, then a slice of tomato, followed by a slice of cheese. Top with an onion slice, squash, and more cheese, finishing with the second slice of eggplant. Insert a metal or wooden skewer through the center of

each stack from top to bottom. Take a stalk of rosemary and trim off bottom leaves. Insert rosemary stalk next to skewer.

4. Bake stacks for about five minutes or until cheese is melted and vegetables are heated through. Transfer stacks to serving plate and carefully pull out skewers.

 TIP: Try serving these stacks on a bed of angel hair pasta with pesto sauce. You can also grill the vegetables instead of roasting them.

 Potato-Cheese Frittata (Serves 2-4)

Serve this frittata warm or at room temperature. It makes a tasty leftover for breakfast or lunch.

Ingredients

2 tsp olive oil

1 small onion, chopped

2 green onions, sliced diagonally

6 cooked small new potatoes, peeled and sliced
   (about 3/4 lb)

3 large eggs

2 large egg whites

2 tbsp low-fat milk

Salt and pepper to taste

3 tbsp shredded Cheddar cheese

Directions

1. In an 8- or 9-inch, non-stick, ovenproof skillet, heat oil over medium heat. Add all onions and cook, stirring occasionally, until softened, about five minutes. Add potatoes to skillet, spreading to cover bottom of the pan.

2. In a medium bowl, whisk together eggs, egg whites, milk, salt, and pepper. Reduce heat to low and pour egg mixture over vegetables, covering evenly. Cover and cook until egg mixture has set around edges but center is still liquid, six to eight minutes.

3. Preheat broiler. Scatter cheese over surface of egg-potato mixture. Place skillet under broiler and cook until lightly golden, about one minute. Cut frittata into four wedges and serve warm.

Barbecuing

Summer holidays are synonymous with grilling. Grilling meat is a steadfast North American tradition, but recent reports suggest that it may not be the most healthful habit for you and your family. Before you fire up that grill, take note of some of the pros and cons of barbecuing.

The positive side is that grilling food is a low-fat way to cook. Grilling is also a quick cooking method that can save time in the kitchen, cutting down on pans to be scrubbed.

The negative side is that grilled foods have a higher potential for carcinogens. Fat that drips onto the flames creates smoke that contains polycyclic aromatic hydrocarbons—chemicals in smoke that are potentially toxic.

Although it's prudent to reduce exposure to these potentially toxic substances as much as possible, I'm sure that having a grilled meal every now and then is not going to kill you. If you love to grill, consider lightly cooking foods first to reduce grilling time. Use low or medium heat on the grill and try to avoid having flames shoot up and char the food. Although the blackened parts taste great, try to avoid eating them, because that's where the suspected carcinogens are.

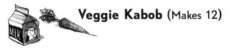 **Veggie Kabob** (Makes 12)

Get ready for this flavorful grilling treat!

Ingredients
1/4 stick butter (or soy margarine)
1/4 cup olive oil
Cilantro
Cayenne pepper
Cumin and garlic (crushed)
2 parboiled potatoes
1 bag miniature bulb onions

2 green peppers

2 red peppers

2 small zucchini

Container cherry tomatoes

6 large mushrooms

2 ears corn

Directions

1. Melt butter in a saucepan. Add olive oil, cilantro, cayenne pepper, cumin, and garlic, to taste. Sauté at low temperature for 10 minutes, but don't boil.

2. Cut vegetables into large pieces (one inch or slightly larger). Pierce vegetables with skewers and place on the grill or broil in the oven.

3. Spoon butter mixture over vegetables each time you turn skewers while grilling.

4. Be careful not to overcook. The veggies should still be a bit crunchy.

TiP: Feel free to use any marinade you want.

Vegan Potato Salad (Serves 4)

This is great for summer picnics and dinners on the deck. Two kinds of potatoes add extra flavor.

Ingredients
4 large Yukon potatoes
2 small red potatoes
1/2 cup Nayonnaise
1/2 cup chopped onion
3/4 cup chopped celery
4 tbsp pickle relish
4 tsp white vinegar
Salt and pepper to taste

Directions
1. Boil potatoes for 25 minutes and then drain. In a separate bowl, combine Nayonnaise, onion, celery, and relish. Mix.
2. When potatoes are cooled, peel Yukon potatoes only (red potatoes should remain in their skins, which add texture to the salad). Cube potatoes and add to Nayonnaise mixture.
3. Add vinegar and salt and pepper, to taste, and then toss.

 TIP: You can always adjust recipe by adding red or green peppers, red onion, different potatoes, et cetera.

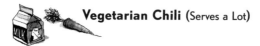 **Vegetarian Chili** (Serves a Lot)

If your barbecue party isn't complete without a big bowl of chili, you'll love this recipe. Try smothering it over a soy dog and watch your child's eyes light up.

Ingredients
2 1/2 cups dry kidney beans

1 tsp salt

1 cup tomato juice

1 cup raw bulgur

1 1/2 cups chopped onions

4 cloves crushed garlic

Olive oil to sauté vegetables

1/2 cup chopped carrots

1 cup chopped celery

1 tsp ground cumin

1 tsp basil

1 tsp chili powder

Dash of cayenne

Salt and pepper to taste

1/2 cup chopped green pepper

2 cups chopped fresh tomatoes

3 tbsp tomato paste

3 tbsp dry red wine

2 tbsp lemon juice

Grated cheese (or soy cheese)

Directions

1. Put kidney beans in a saucepan and cover them with six cups of water. Soak overnight. Add extra water and one teaspoon of salt and cook until tender—about one hour. Add more water if necessary as the beans are cooking.
2. Heat tomato juice to a boil and pour over raw bulgur. Cover and let stand for 15 minutes.
3. Sauté onions and garlic in olive oil. Add carrots, celery, and spices. When vegetables are almost cooked, add peppers. Cook for about two more minutes.
4. Combine all ingredients and heat together. Adjust seasoning to taste and serve sprinkled with cheese.

Happy Birthday to You

No celebration is attended more frequently by young people than the birthday party. These occasions can be hard for vegetarians. But when it comes time for your child's birthday, have no fear—vegan cakes are tasty and easy to make.

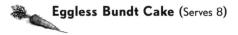 **Eggless Bundt Cake** (Serves 8)

You won't be able to wait until the candles are blown out to dig into this light and sumptuous cake topped with a decadent fudge frosting.

Ingredients

1 1/2 cups pastry flour

1 1/2 cups unbleached white flour

1 1/2 tbsp baking powder

1/2 tsp sea salt

1/2 cup safflower oil

1 cup maple syrup

1 1/2 cups soy milk

1 tbsp vanilla

Directions

1. Preheat the oven to 350 degrees. Brush a Bundt pan with oil.
2. In a large bowl, mix first four ingredients well. In a medium bowl, whisk remaining ingredients together. Add the wet ingredients into the dry. Whisk just until batter is entirely smooth, being careful not to overmix, which toughens the texture. Pour batter into the pan.
3. Bake about 40 minutes, until cake looks golden on top and is springy to the touch. A toothpick inserted into the center should come out clean. Let cake cool completely at room temperature before frosting.

Frosting Ingredients

1/2 cup vegan margarine

2/3 cup cocoa

3 cups powdered sugar

1/3 cup vanilla soy milk

1 tsp vanilla extract

Directions

1. Melt margarine in a small saucepan. Stir in cocoa.
2. Alternately add powdered sugar and milk, beating at medium speed to spread consistency. Add more milk if needed. Add vanilla.
3. Set aside and let stand until completely cool. When cool, frost cake and let frosting set for an hour. Decorate and voilà!

 TIP: Remember, this cake can be decorated with anything from raisins to vegan "M&M's." Use red and blue berries for July 4th, Reese's Pieces for Halloween, cinnamon hearts for Valentine's Day . . . use your imagination!

 Eggless Butterscotch Chocolate Brownies
(Makes 12-18)

When birthday cake alone isn't enough!

Ingredients

4 oz butter, melted
1 1/2 cups graham cracker crumbs
1 cup walnuts, coarsely chopped
1 cup (6 oz) chocolate chips
1 cup (6 oz) butterscotch chips
1 1/3 cups (3 1/2 oz) flaked coconut
1 1/3 cups (15 oz can) sweetened condensed milk

Directions

1. Pour melted butter into 9- by 13-inch baking pan.
2. Layer remaining ingredients evenly in the order listed.
3. Bake for 25 minutes at 350 degrees or until lightly browned. Cut into squares whatever size you want!

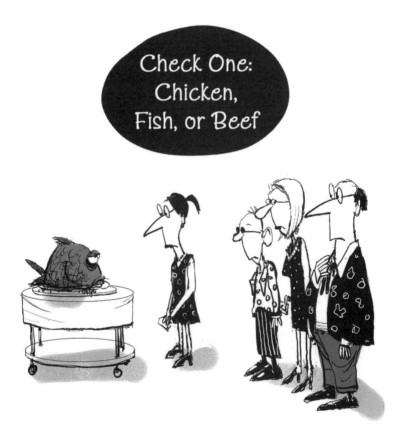

CHAPTER 6

Check One:
Chicken,
Fish, or Beef

Vegetarian Etiquette for You and Your Child

Several years ago, my husband and I were invited to a dinner party at the home of a friend who not only loves to entertain but also offers her cooking as her artistic expression. The table was set with an elegance to which Martha Stewart would have given accolades. The appetizers were exquisite and the salad scrumptious. The main course of Cornish hen surrounded by crab apples sprinkled with walnut chips was, well, let's just say there was no doubt in my mind that our hostess had spent more than a little time lovingly arranging each plate.

As we oohed and aahed over the delicate sauce and the surprise of saffron rice and dried cranberries inside each hen, it appeared that one couple was not sharing in our delight. They seemed to be moving the crab apples around a bit and nibbling at the walnuts, but they certainly weren't diving in.

As we all tried to lightly suggest that they begin to eat and joked about how they must have "eaten on the plane," they eventually shared with the hostess that they were sorry, but they didn't eat Cornish hen. "We're vegetarians," they offered. The table fell into awkward silence.

Here is a quiz. If you were the hostess, would you

1. apologize for not being psychic and knowing to prepare something they could have eaten;
2. laugh, say, "That's fine," and make light of the situation;
3. burst into tears; or
4. grab them by the shirt collars, stick a fork in the hen, hold it in front of their faces, and say, "Listen, buddies, I worked all day on these things, and you better eat 'em or else"?

The correct answer is "None of the above" — because this scenario should never have happened. Any vegetarian worth his or her weight in tofu should practice the basic conventions of etiquette, which certainly include informing your hostess that you don't eat meat well before her trip to the butcher.

When Your Child Is Invited Out

Your job as the parent of a vegetarian is not only to make sure that the hostess is informed of your child's food preferences but also to put her at ease and to minimize her efforts to accommodate your child. This seems to be so self-evident, and, had I not been a guest at the aforementioned dinner, I might not have included this chapter.

When your child receives an invitation, you or he should simply call the host and say, "I really don't want to inconvenience you, but I want you to know that Johnny is a vegetarian. Please don't make anything special for him. He's very happy to eat around any meat you may be serving." Usually the host will insist on preparing something special, since most people don't believe that the appetizers, salad, vegetable, starch, and dessert will fill someone up. However, it's your choice, knowing the player, to either graciously accept the offer of a special dish prepared for your child or further insist that she not go to any trouble. If you agree to the offer of a special dish, explain *precisely* what your child will and will not eat—you'd be surprised what some people think constitutes a vegetarian meal. Another option is to offer to send your child with a dish that you've prepared. In either case, at least there won't be any unhappy surprises.

Likewise, when your family receives a written invitation to a wedding or other catered event and the food choice is chicken, beef, or fish, it's up to you to write a gracious note requesting a vegetarian entrée. This type of request is common these days and will make your hostess much happier than throwing away a $100/plate salmon dinner.

Your Curious Friends

Like it or not, part of your job as the parent of a vegetarian is explaining to others why your child has chosen this lifestyle. If you think that your friends and family are going to react by saying, "How proud you must be of Johnny for not wanting to kill innocent animals," or, "You must be a fabulous parent to have a child that cares that much about her health she's willing to

give up meat before her arteries are 98 percent blocked,"
you're in for quite a surprise. It's been 32 years since I've eaten
red meat, and it continues to amaze me how normally well-man-
nered people can lose all sense of propriety when this subject
comes up. Reactions vacillate between

1. *nonexpressed hostility* (watch for the almost unde-
   tectable roll of the eyes);
2. *sympathy* ("I know what you must be going through.
   My sister's son pulled that one on her too"); and
3. *accusations of ulterior motives* ("What do you think
   he's trying to prove?").

I recommend that you, as his parent, defend his choice.

Your child's decision to become a vegetarian can cause
disharmony and division not only in your immediate family but
in your extended family as well. Remember, your child is going
to have to endure teasing, challenging questions, and outright
rudeness from both friends and strangers for perhaps the rest
of his life. How great it would be if he could count on you for
unwavering support.

You can use several different responses when called upon
to defend your child's decision. Pick the one that suits you the
best.

1. *Be straightforward and honest* about why your child made
   the decision to become a vegetarian: "Diane loves animals
   very much, and she just chose to no longer eat anything

that has a face," or, "Katherine has decided that being a vegetarian is more in line with her beliefs about nonviolence, and I'm supportive of her decision."

2. *Give a helpful answer* that might provide the curious with food for thought: "I'm actually quite pleased with Antoine's decision. I can see now that he is going to grow up with a much greater chance of not getting heart disease and cancer, and that makes me very happy."

3. *Ask them to join you in giving your child support:* "You know, it's not easy being a vegetarian in a meat-eating world. Why don't you join me in being supportive of Justin? He's made up his mind, and his father and I have decided that nothing positive can come from resisting or belittling his decision."

4. *Use "feel, felt, found."* Some people become confrontational because they feel that their own lifestyle choices are being questioned. You can assuage this fear with the old technique of "feel, felt, found." It helps people to know that you are not judging their choice to eat meat. It works like this. Let's say someone says to you, "I knew a woman whose daughter became anorexic from being a vegetarian." Instead of saying "That's totally ridiculous. People don't become anorexic from being vegetarians," say, "I know absolutely why you would *feel* that way. When Judy first told me that she was going to be a vegetarian, I *felt* that maybe

she was developing some eating disorder. But now I've *found* that. . . ." This approach is the most helpful when you are dealing with self-proclaimed experts, adamant carnivores, and those who, for whatever reason, have something against tempeh.

One last point to remember: no apologies necessary.

Your Child's Own Responsibility

Have you ever heard the expression "There's no one worse than an ex-smoker"? That may have been true in the past, but now I've found someone worse—a new vegetarian. Some can be incorrigibly self-righteous.

Several years ago, the teenage daughter of a friend of mine decided that she was no longer going to eat meat. And she decided that it was time for everyone else on the planet to change their eating habits too. Being a good-natured sort, I found it humorous when, over dinner one night, she started lecturing me on the level of mercury in my whitefish. But my humor quickly turned to abhorrence when she felt compelled to inform the other guests, happily enjoying their chicken Marsala, that up to 25 percent of slaughtered chickens on the inspection line are covered with feces, bile, and feed.

Part of your agreement with your vegetarian child should be that you will be respectful of her choice if she is respectful of yours and others'. Of course, this doesn't mean that she can't share her unique ideas and feelings, but the key here is *respect*. If we become convinced that only our way is right, and we don't respect others' choices, then we're all in trouble. If she really wants others to adopt a vegetarian lifestyle, then she shouldn't deride their food choices. If she does, then she will certainly get the opposite result.

Recently my daughter came home from school ranting about how stupid vegetarians are. Surprised at her adamancy, I asked what had happened, and it turned out that some new vegetarians had done the "yuck" thing over her best friend's bologna sandwich at lunch. That had been enough to make her swear she'd never be a strict vegetarian again.

Respect and timing are the cornerstones of etiquette, vegetarian or otherwise.

CHAPTER 7

Can We Still Go out for Dinner?

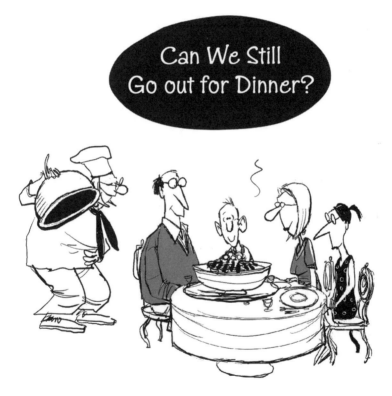

From Moo Shoo to Manicotti, You Can Still Dine Out

In the late 1970s, I was the director of admissions at a small liberal arts college in southeast Iowa. My assistant and I, both strict vegetarians, were invited to participate in a two-day workshop in Fort Dodge. We had some concerns about what we would eat since this was not only the 1970s but also the pork capital of America. We figured that we wouldn't die even if we ate only iceberg lettuce and canned green beans for two days. Imagine our surprise when we sat down to order our first meal at the restaurant in the Best Western Hotel and there on the menu was "vegetarian burger."

We felt a little bad about all the pork jokes and thought that we owed Iowa an apology as we sat and eagerly anticipated the arrival of our dinner. Imagine our even greater surprise when those "vegetarian burgers" arrived and we lifted the buns to find two juicy beef patties topped with lettuce, tomato, and a pickle.

Times have changed. What a difference a quarter of a century makes! Most menus now have a section labeled "Vegetarian Entrées"—not only in Santa Cruz and Berkeley but also in Houston and Fort Dodge—and even Burger King now offers a veggie burger.

So don't worry, Mom and Dad, you can still take the kids out for dinner from sea to shining sea. But to completely alleviate lingering doubts about your child being able to get something to eat, I'll give you my "Best Bet" options, and you can choose where you want to go.

Best Bet 1: Chinese/Thai/Vietnamese

Most Asian restaurants now include tofu dishes and even some selections with seitan. If they don't, there are still plenty of dishes full of nutritious vegetables, grains, and even nuts and legumes such as cashews and peanuts. Try vegetable egg rolls or spring rolls for appetizers. From the moo shoo vegetables or vegetable pad thai to the egg foo yung for the lacto-ovos, you will find more than enough to satisfy any vegetarian's hunger. Just remember to ask for no MSG or fish sauce.

Best Bet 2: Italian

The problem with an Italian restaurant is that there are too many choices! Even if you are a vegan, there's a big Italian salad with all the trimmings. For everyone else, the sky's the limit with pasta primavera, pasta marinara, yummy pesto sauce, vegetarian pizza, cheese ravioli, mushroom tortellini, eggplant Parmigiana, pasta Alfredo, cheesy manicotti, or vegetarian lasagna. And don't forget the garlic bread and the sweet ricotta calzones! Yum!

Best Bet 3: Mexican

Mexican restaurants are mostly about rice, beans, and salsa served 101 different ways. Add the cheese and you have 201. At our favorite little Mexican café, we start out with chips dipped in guacamole and salsa, move on to the tortilla soup, and then stuff ourselves with gigantic vegetable, black bean, and avocado burritos, while the fish eaters indulge in the fish tacos, and the younger children eat bean and cheese tostadas. For those who eat eggs, some favorites are the chile rellenos or huevos rancheros. And for dessert, well, what's a Mexican meal without flan? Or for the strict vegetarians, there are always sopapillas.

Best Bet 4: Middle Eastern

In my early twenties, I spent several months living in Israel. Let me tell you, the Middle East is a vegetarian's paradise. Instead of serving hot dogs and hamburgers, the corner joints and street vendors all sell falafels overflowing with fried chickpea balls, lettuce, tomatoes, and tahini dressing. It's more common to see children eating cucumber salad from a cup than it is to see them eating French fries. People pop grape leaves stuffed with couscous or tiny spinach pies in their mouths more often than M & M's. And all these vegetarian delights, as well as hummus on pita bread and savory eggplant baba ghanoush, are waiting for you at your local Middle Eastern restaurant.

Best Bet 5: Indian

I love Indian food, and, if it weren't a bit exotic (and spicy) for most young people, I'd put it as Best Bet 1. The variety is endless since many Indian people, for religious reasons, are vegetarian.

Appetizer choices include vegetable samosa, a flaky golden pasty stuffed with potatoes, green peas, and spices, and vegetable pakora, the Indian equivalent of tempura. Main courses include everything from spinach and paneer (deep-fried cheese cubes) to baigan bharta (fresh eggplant roasted and mashed with herbs and spices). My favorites are aloo gobhi (cauliflower and potatoes sautéed with tomatoes, onion, garlic, ginger, herbs, and spices) and tandoori vegetables, roasted in a clay oven. Entrées are typically served with basmati rice, often flavored with saffron, and exotic breads such as naan, baked in the tandoori oven. Be sure to leave room for the out-of-this-world variety of sweets, including halwa and kulfi (traditional Indian ice cream).

Best Bet 6: Japanese

Once again, since we are talking about taking our children out for dinner, I don't want to get too carried away with my favorites. Japanese food can be heavy on the seaweed and raw fish, which can sometimes be a bit much for some young people. However, if your kids are daring in the eating department, then they should give Japanese food a try. Start out with vegetable tempura and a bowl of edamame (boiled soybeans in the pods). Although it sounds a bit lackluster, it's really very delicious. My daughter loves vegetarian "maki rolls," which come with cucumbers, avocados, shitake mushrooms, spinach, carrots, or all of the above rolled in rice and seaweed. Japanese restaurants also have excellent noodle dishes. Try soba (buckwheat) noodles or udon (white flour) noodles mixed with vegetables and tofu.

Best Bet 7: If You Have to Go to a Steak Joint

There are plenty of things for any vegetarian to eat even at a steak joint. I've yet to see an appetizer list that doesn't include cheese quesadillas, hot artichoke dip, deep-fried mushrooms, or stuffed potato skins (just make sure the cooks leave off the bacon bits—if they're real, which usually they aren't). Pick two or three appetizers, and you have a meal! And even if there aren't special vegetarian entrées, not only are some of the best salads in town found at these establishments (try the Caesar without anchovies), but also they usually have great vegetables and even greater potatoes—a big baked potato stuffed with veggies and melted cheese is a very filling main course for a vegetarian and something that any steak house should be happy to prepare for your child.

Living in a Fast-Food World

In 1974, I was the event coordinator for a large conference taking place at a convention facility in the suburbs of Chicago. It was the night before the event, and at two in the morning we were still setting up the stage, arranging flowers, collating materials, and getting a little hungry. So we decided that three of us would go on a search for an all-night restaurant and bring food back for the rest of the group. The search became even more of a challenge since we were all vegetarians.

After driving for quite a while, we spied the Golden Arches in the distance like celestial lights and pulled into the parking lot. No problem, we'd been there before, and we knew exactly what we wanted. So we walked up to the friendly order taker and told him "We'll have six Big Macs, hold the meat, six fries, and six root beers." After a long silent pause, he looked up, eyes wide, and asked, "Did you say what I think you said?" So we clearly repeated our order as he slowly turned around and called out to the man behind the stove, "You won't believe this one! They want six Big Macs, *hold the meat,* six fries, and six root beers." As the man in the back craned his neck to see what we looked like, our order taker turned back to us and with all sincerity asked, "Are you sure this ain't *Candid Camera?*"

Fast-forward to 2003. Although there's nothing wrong with a Big Mac, hold the meat (just a fabulous cheese, lettuce, tomato, pickle, and onion sandwich on a sesame seed bun), vegetarians now have as many fast-food choices as their meat-eating friends. I'm not claiming any great health benefits from fast food, but sometimes the pace of contemporary life makes a stop at the drive thru unavoidable. My vegetarian favorites include

- vegetarian sandwiches at Subway and Quiznos;
- cheese pizza at Pizza Hut;
- corn on the cob, baked beans, potato wedges, and coleslaw at KFC;
- veggie burgers at Burger King (or Whoppers with cheese, hold the meat);
- seven-layer burritos at Taco Bell (or any combination of beans, cheese, veggies, and rice at any quick Mexican food chain);

- salads at McDonald's;
- salad bar and salad pockets at Wendy's; and
- "3 Sides Sampler" at Boston Market (try the creamed spinach and the sweet potatoes or, for fewer grams of fat, the green beans or vegetable medley).

Although there's nothing like Mom or Dad's cooking to warm the soul of your child, there are times when you feel like piling the family into the car and heading out for some dining adventure—and now you know that, even with a vegetarian living under your roof, you can still go out for dinner.

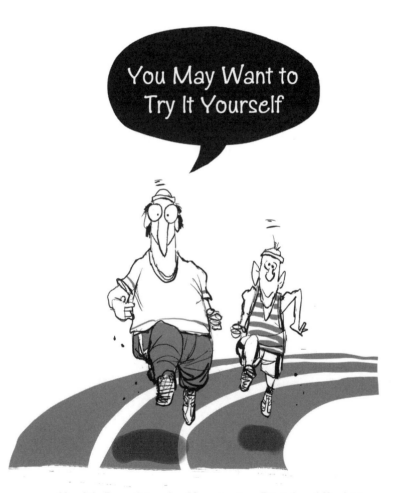

CHAPTER 8

Health Benefits of a Vegetarian Diet for All of Us

It isn't unusual these days that the lifestyle choices we make are inspired by our children. Although my daughter is only 15, I find myself reading books that she recommends, sticking to my own exercise routine to keep up with her unwavering commitment to fitness, and examining many choices that I've made in my life when she shares with me how they look from her perspective. I'm no longer surprised when told by many adults that they themselves became vegetarians as a direct result of having to accommodate their vegetarian children.

The Surgeon General and the American Dietetic Association Can't Both Be Wrong

Former surgeon general C. Everett Koop stated that "70 percent of all Americans are dying from diseases that are directly tied to their eating habits." According to the ADA, diabetes, cardiovascular disease, hypertension, cancer, and gastrointestinal problems can all develop as direct results of our food choices. Saturated fat, cholesterol, and high-calorie foods are literally killing us.

Unfortunately too many people don't think enough about the negative long-term effects of their food choices. They keep on eating hamburgers and fries and drinking shakes, feeling confident that advanced medical procedures can clean out arteries as easily as a dentist can clean your teeth. It's really not as easy, or free of risk, as you may think. But what is easy and risk free is preventing illness with proper nutrition — paying equal attention to what you should eat and what you shouldn't.

Adopting a vegetarian or vegan diet will maximize your chances of health and longevity and minimize your chances of developing many 21st century diseases. The right diet might even restore ideal health to an ailing person.

According to a study from Loma Linda University, vegetarians live about seven years longer than meat eaters. This finding is backed by the China Health Project, the most extensive study on diet and health to date, which found that people who eat the least amount of fat and animal products have the lowest risks of cancer, heart attack, and other chronic degenerative diseases. Furthermore, a British study that tracked 6,000 vegetarians and 5,000 meat eaters for 12 years found that vegetarians were 40 percent less likely to die from cancer during that time and 20 percent less likely to die from other diseases.

Many doctors now believe that a plant-based diet is the "wonder cure" of the 21st century. "There's no question that largely vegetarian diets are as healthy as you can get," states

Marion Nestle, chair of the Department of Nutrition at New York University. "The evidence is so strong and overwhelming and produced over such a long period of time that it's no longer debatable."

The Disease-Fighting Power of Vegetarian Diets

Populations around the world with a large percentage of vegetarians generally enjoy unusually good health, characterized by low rates of cancer and cardiovascular disease as well as lower cholesterol levels, blood pressure, and total mortality. Why?

There are a number of biological reasons a vegetarian diet slows or prevents the onset of chronic diseases. Vegetables and fruits are rich sources of vitamins, trace minerals, and dietary fiber. Hidden inside these nutrients are two protective substances: antioxidants and phytochemicals. Scientists believe that these are the gems of good health and preventive medicine.

Antioxidants

You've likely heard the term "antioxidant" but may not know what it means. Antioxidants are a family of nutrients with proven disease-fighting powers. The most well-studied antioxidants are household names, such as vitamin E, vitamin C, beta- carotene, folic acid, and the mineral selenium, although scientists think that the most powerful antioxidants yet discovered are found in grape seed extract. Antioxidants have an uncanny ability to disarm free radicals.

Free radicals are oxygen molecules with a missing or unpaired electron that spin erratically throughout the body, damaging cells and tissue that they come in contact with until they are stopped by an antioxidant. Free radicals destroy cell membranes, damage collagen, disrupt important physiological processes, and even create mutations in the DNA of cells. Free radicals are known to cause premature aging, heart disease, atherosclerosis, cancer, and a host of other degenerative conditions, including Alzheimer's, cataracts, and arthritis. Free radicals are produced to a degree by normal body metabolism but are mostly a result of exposure to toxic chemicals in the environment, radiation, certain drugs, alcohol, saturated fats, cigarette smoke, pesticides in our foods, additives, preservatives, and colorants.

Scientists believe that many common diseases can be prevented if people adopt diets rich in antioxidants. Fruits and vegetables—notably citrus fruits, dark green and red vegetables, vegetables such as sweet potatoes and carrots, as well as whole wheat, oatmeal, rye, nuts, and all grains—grown in selenium-rich soil are excellent sources of antioxidants.

Phytochemicals

Vegetarian diets are also rich in phytochemicals. The term "phytochemicals" means chemicals found in plants. They give a plant its color, flavor, and smell and are part of a plant's natural defense system. It is the defensive qualities in phytochemicals that have researchers intrigued, because the same qualities may also benefit humans.

Like their antioxidant brethren, phytochemicals have impressive disease-fighting résumés. Researchers believe that phytochemicals could go a long way in helping reduce the risk of several chronic diseases, including heart disease and cancer.

Numerous studies have already linked phytochemicals to the prevention and treatment of heart disease, diabetes, and high blood pressure. Phytochemicals also support immune functions and combat tumors and viruses. A number of phytochemicals are known to interfere with the cancer process by preventing carcinogens from forming. Although research in this field is still in its beginning stage, hundreds of phytochemicals have been identified, including 40 in broccoli, 50 in garlic and onions, 70 in the herb tarragon, and more than 170 in oranges. Most fruits and vegetables are phytochemical gold mines. Brightly colored fruits and vegetables — yellow, orange, red, green, blue, and purple — generally contain the most phytochemicals and the most nutrients. Increasing your phytochemical consumption is a great way to improve your health.

Specific Diseases Affected by a Vegetarian Diet

Asthma

In his groundbreaking book *Diet for a New America*, John Robbins notes that 90 percent of asthma patients put on a completely vegetarian diet (without meat, eggs, or dairy products) experienced great improvements in the frequency and severity of their asthma attacks. The greatest improvement was shown by those who eliminated dairy products. Unfortunately most asthmatics aren't aware of the many published studies showing that high dietary intake of dairy aggravates asthma.

Andrew Weil, author of *Optimum Wellness*, also advises asthma patients to eliminate milk and milk products, substituting other calcium sources. He also advises them to decrease protein to 10 percent of daily caloric intake and to replace animal protein with plant protein. Consuming fruits and vegetables is recommended for asthmatics because vitamin C creates an antihistamine response. Additionally, when foods rich in vitamin C are consumed with foods rich in the B-complex vitamins, the balanced production of epinephrine and norepinephrine will reduce bronchial constriction. Bioflavonoids, such as those found in red grapes, are also potent antihistamines.

Cardiovascular Disease

As heart expert Ann Japenga notes, heart disease—not cancer—is the number one killer in North America. Approximately 57 million Americans—nearly one in four—have one or more types of cardiovascular disease, and 955,000 die of it each year—or 2,600 every day. In one year alone, the number of people who die of heart attacks equals the number of American soldiers who would have died in 10 Vietnam Wars. The typical American diet, laden with saturated fat and cholesterol from meat and dairy, is largely to blame. According to the Bogalusa Heart Study conducted at Louisiana State University, children raised on fast food and junk food show early signs of heart disease at as young as three years old.

Today the average American male eating a meat-based diet has a 50 percent chance of dying from heart disease. His risk drops to 35 percent if he cuts out meat and to four percent if he cuts out meat, dairy, and eggs. Heart disease is caused not by meat but by the fat and cholesterol meat contributes to your diet. Dietary fat, saturated in particular, has been shown to be the main culprit in heart disease.

Compared with nonvegetarians, vegetarians suffer markedly lower mortality from the most common form of cardiovascular disease, called coronary heart disease. Findings from the Oxford Vegetarian Study, a 12-year study of 6,000 vegetarians and 5,000 meat eaters, found that the incidence of coronary heart disease mortality was 28 percent lower in vegetarians compared with matched meat eaters. As reported by J. Claude-Chang, an 11-year study of 1,900 German vegetarians echoed this result, finding mortality from cardiovascular disease to be 61 percent lower in male vegetarians and 44 percent lower in female vegetarians than in the general population.

Cholesterol

According to famed heart researcher Dean Ornish, a low-fat vegetarian diet together with other lifestyle changes such as exercise and stress management can in fact reverse the progress of heart disease by reducing cholesterol plaques in coronary arteries.

Cholesterol is a waxy substance found in all parts of the body. It helps to form cell membranes as well as vitamin D and hormones. Some cholesterol is made inside the body, and some comes from dietary sources such as dairy, meat, and egg yolks. Since your liver makes all the cholesterol that your body needs, too much from your diet can make LDL ("bad") cholesterol levels rise too high and damage arteries. Once they are damaged, the cholesterol can continue to build up, and eventually those arteries can block the flow of blood to the heart, resulting in a heart attack, or to the brain, resulting in a stroke.

To lower your level of LDL cholesterol, cut saturated fats and dietary cholesterol, and eat foods high in fiber, specifically vegetables, fruits, and whole grains.

Hypertension (High Blood Pressure)

A startling statistic in the May 4, 1999, edition of the *New York Times* revealed that only 18 percent of people with high blood pressure are successfully treated to achieve normal ranges. Untreated, hypertension carries enormous health risks, such as increased risk of heart disease, stroke, kidney disease, and eye disease. High blood pressure also causes the arteries and arterioles to become scarred, hardened, and less elastic. This damage, in turn, can limit the amount of blood flowing to the organs, cause blood clots in the arteries, and ultimately damage the heart, brain, and kidneys.

In 95 percent of cases, hypertension is related to lifestyle factors such as body weight, lack of exercise, smoking, excessive alcohol consumption, and diet. Hypertension is treated in three ways: prescription medication, diet, and lifestyle changes.

A 1996 Harvard University study of 41,541 female nurses, published in *Hypertension Journal*, concluded that "a diet rich in fruits and vegetables may reduce blood pressure levels." In addition, according to the American Dietetic Association's position on vegetarian diets, as reported in the *Journal of the American Dietetic Association*, "Vegetarians tend to have a lower incidence of hypertension than nonvegetarians. This effect appears to be *independent* of both weight and sodium intake."

Cancer

As noted by R. Doll of the Nutrition Society, diet may be linked to 30 – 70 percent of cancers. Nick Day of Cambridge University and the European Prospective Study into Cancer stated that "Vegetarians may suffer 40% fewer cancers than the general population."

According to the American Cancer Society, more than 500,000 people die from cancer each year in the United States, roughly half of them women. Many medical practitioners are now beginning to stress to their patients the importance of eating a plant-centered diet to reduce the risk of developing cancer. Experts now agree that many plant foods contain substances that can help us to avoid cancer and that a low-fat, plant-based diet can slow or reverse tumor growth and bolster the body's natural resistance to disease.

One such substance is resveratrol, found abundantly in grape skins. John Pezzuto, the leader of a food research group at the University of Illinois in Chicago working with cell cultures and laboratory animals, has found that resveratrol can keep cells from turning cancerous and inhibit the spread of cells already malignant. Pezzuto, the senior author of a study published in the journal *Science*, said that his group conducted hundreds of tests looking for anticancer compounds in foods widely available and non-toxic. Although many fruits and vegetables exhibited natural chemopreventive activity, Michael Wargovich, a cancer researcher at M.D. Anderson Hospital in Houston, said that resveratrol "really hits a home run in the range of activity it has against cancer. However, my advice would be not to rely on grapes alone. This is just one part of the fruit and vegetable story."

Breast cancer is the second most commonly diagnosed cancer in the United States, striking 182,000 women each year and killing more than 46,000. A study in the *International Journal of Cancer* concluded that red meat is strongly associated with breast cancer. And the National Cancer Institute says that women who eat meat every day are nearly four times more likely to develop breast cancer than those who don't. "We have consistent evidence that an affluent, Western diet is associated with higher risk of breast cancer," says Regina Ziegler, a nutritional epidemiologist at the National Cancer Institute. "Breast cancer is essentially a dietary disease, just as lung cancer is essentially a smoking-related disease," says Dr. Robert Kradjian, a breast surgeon for nearly 30 years and the author of *Save Yourself from Breast Cancer*. He adds, "If you want to avoid breast cancer, then learn to live like the billions of women on this earth who will avoid the disease. Eat a diet high in protective vegetables, fruits, and fiber—a plant-based diet."

Studies have also found that a plant-based diet helps to protect against prostate, colon, and skin cancers. "The science base is very strong that fruits and vegetables are protective for all the gastrointestinal cancers and all smoking related cancers," says Tim Byers, a professor of preventive medicine at the University of Colorado Health Sciences Center in Denver. The link between a meat-centered diet and the high incidence of colon cancer is nearly irrefutable. International studies suggest that fully 95 percent of colon cancer cases have a connection to nutrition. In 1992, as reported in the *Journal of the National Cancer Institute*, researchers found that women who ate about six to 10 servings of fruits and vegetables per day had a 38 percent lower risk of fatal colon cancer than women who ate the least number of servings. In one study involving more than 88,000 women, researchers found that those who ate the most animal fat were nearly twice as likely to develop colon cancer as those who ate the least animal fat. Quoted by Gina Kolata, study director Walter Willet concluded that, "If you step back and look at the data, the optimum amount of red meat you eat should be zero."

Osteoporosis

Osteoporosis affects more than 20 million American women. This disease is responsible for the loss of bone tissue that weakens bones and heightens the likelihood of fracture. It is known that bone health and osteoporosis are also closely linked to diet.

The average bone loss for a vegetarian woman at age 65 is 18 percent; for nonvegetarian women, it's double that (see www.melhuish.org/vegetarian.htm). Researchers have attributed this loss to the consumption of excess protein. The average meat-eating American woman consumes 144 percent over the recommended daily allowance; the average man consumes 175 percent more. Excess protein in the diet actually interferes with the absorption and retention of calcium and prompts the body to excrete calcium, laying the ground for brittle bones. This excretion occurs because animal proteins, including milk, make the blood acidic. The body pulls calcium from the bones to balance that condition. Thus, dark green leafy vegetables and legumes seem to be, calorie for calorie, superior sources of calcium.

A number of top researchers believe that calcium loss is more important to overall calcium balance than how much of the mineral we consume. "Logic may tell us that calcium intake ought to be important, but the evidence is weak," says Mark Hegsted, a highly respected calcium researcher from Harvard University (as cited by Judy Krizmanic). Christiane Northrup notes that Hegsted's conclusion is supported by numerous studies showing that "Eating a balanced, mostly vegetarian diet rich in greens such as kale, collards and broccoli is the first step to prevent calcium loss." To fight the onset of osteoporosis, it's important not only to increase calcium but also to decrease meat in your diet.

Diabetes

The incidence of Type II diabetes, also called adult onset diabetes, is skyrocketing worldwide. Approximately eight percent of American adults have been diagnosed with this condition, and many more are living with it undiagnosed.

Although millions of dollars are being poured into research, so far there hasn't been a medication developed that returns blood sugar levels to normal or eliminates common diabetic complications, such as blindness, heart attack, and kidney failure. Treatment with diet, however, has been found to reduce these symptoms for a lifetime.

Diabetes is aggravated by a diet full of fat and deficient in plant foods. The association between fat and diabetes has been accepted in the medical community for over 75 years. In 1927, Dr. E.P. Joslin, founder of the famous Joslin Diabetic Center in Boston, suspected that a high-fat, high-cholesterol diet might lead to the development of diabetes and its major complication, atherosclerosis.

A study published in the February 2002 *Annals of Internal Medicine*, which included 51,529 male health professionals, found that those whose diets were rich in red meat, high-fat dairy products, and baked goods were 60 percent more likely to develop diabetes than those who ate a diet consisting predominantly of vegetables, fruits, and whole grains. Obese subjects had more than 11 times the risk of developing diabetes.

Conclusion

As you can see, there is strong evidence that a vegetarian diet can be a powerful stepping-stone toward optimum health for your vegetarian child and your entire family. With such an abundance of research pointing to the superiority of a vegetarian diet, you just may want to try it yourself.

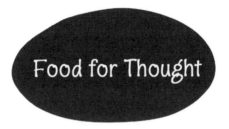

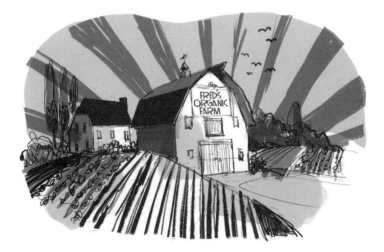

CHAPTER 9

Lesser-Known Facts about the Food We Eat

In this chapter, I will share with you some lesser-known facts about what is in our food supply. Because of the seriousness of this issue, it's difficult to continue in a lighthearted vein. However, as long as you're making some changes in your household, with this additional information in hand, you may choose to go the extra mile and start paying even closer attention to what you are feeding your family. My intent is not to be political or to scare you, but I believe that many of you want to know the information that follows so that you can make your own informed decisions about what goes onto your plate. For your sake, for the sake of your family, and for the future of the planet, I don't want to pretend that these issues don't exist, and I don't think you do either.

Organic versus Non-Organic

In September 2002, the cover of *Newsweek* magazine pictured a big apple with the headline "Should You Buy Organic?" Although the writer's intent was evidently to give a balanced assessment of organic versus non-organic foods, the underlying message of the article was clear: organic is better—not only for you but for our planet as well.

In just two years, between 1998 and 2000, sales of organic fruits and vegetables increased by 23 percent, sales of organic meats by 71 percent, and sales of organic grains by a whopping 99 percent. In 2001 alone, sales of organic foods generated $11 billion in the United States, and organic production is now the fastest-growing sector of agriculture. But many people have questions: Is organic food more nutritious than conventional food? Is it worth the additional cost? And what does the term "organic" mean anyway?

Organic food differs from conventionally produced food in the way that it is grown, handled, and processed. Unlike conventional produce, all products sold as "organic" must be certified. The label "certified organic" refers to agricultural products that have been grown and processed according to uniform standards and verified by independent state or private organizations accredited by the USDA. In October 2002, the National Organic Rule went into effect in the United States: any food labeled as "organic" must be produced without hormones, antibiotics, herbicides, insecticides, chemical fertilizers, genetic modification, or germ-killing radiation. Rather than a different set of organic standards in each state, there is now a uniform set of organic production, processing, and labeling standards across the United States (see www.ams.usda.gov/nop).

The USDA makes no claim that organically produced food is better than conventionally produced food. Yet, according to a study done by the Hartman Group of Bellevue, Washington, 38 percent of the respondents said that the flavors of organic fruits and vegetables were clearly superior. "The difference is huge," said Peter Hoffman, owner of New York's Restaurant Savoy when asked why he chooses organic fruits and vegetables. "When people taste asparagus and string beans grown in richly composted soil, they can't get over the depth and vibrancy of the flavor."

Pesticides

Flavor is only one reason people choose organic foods, and it's not the most compelling reason. A 2002 report authored by B.P. Baker and Associates indicates that organic food is far less likely to contain pesticide residues than conventional food. Only 13 percent of organic produce samples versus 71 percent of conventional produce samples contained residues of one or more, and often as many as 10, pesticides. According to homemaker Wendy Abrams, quoted in *Newsweek* in September 2002, "When you buy an apple that has poison on it, even if you wash it, you don't know how much has really come off." She, like other health-conscious parents, has common sense on her side, especially since children, because of their size, consume pesticide residues in much higher proportions than adults.

A report released by the Environmental Working Group entitled *Pesticides in Children's Food* concluded that the largest contribution to a person's lifetime risk of cancer from pesticide residues occurs during childhood. This group provoked protests from agri-industry trade groups when it published findings from a study conducted on a group of insecticides known as organophosphates, derivatives of nerve gases developed in Nazi Germany. The group found that over 1.1 million children under the age of five eat food that contains an unsafe dose of one or more organophosphates—*every day*. Of them, 106,000 children exceeded the FDA's safe daily dosage by 10 times or more. Dr. Herbert L. Needleman, a University of Pittsburgh professor of pediatrics and psychology, warns that "These chemicals do affect the brain and the nervous system, and [children's] developing nervous systems are more vulnerable. Certain pesticides that are highly concentrated should be banned."

According to the EPA and a 1987 National Academy of Science report, laboratory studies show that pesticides can cause birth defects, nerve damage, cancer, and disruptions to the immune system. Farmers consistently exposed to pesticides have an 80 percent higher rate of prostate cancer and increased male infertility.

Pesticides on our food are not only toxic but have also been found to block the absorption of other nutrients necessary for normal healthy growth. The foods most likely to contain unsafe levels of pesticides are peaches, nectarines, strawberries, grapes, apples, pears, and raisins—all popular children's foods.

More Nutritious

If you aren't already convinced to buy organic foods, consider that organic produce packs in more nutrition bite per bite. A recently published review of 41 scientific studies from countries around the world comparing the nutrition of organic and conventionally grown foods found significantly higher nutrients in organic crops. The review, published in the *Journal of Alternative and Complementary Medicine*, notes that such crops, on average, contained 29.3 percent more magnesium, 27 percent more vitamin C, 21 percent more iron, 13.6 percent more phosphorus, 26 percent more calcium, 11 percent more copper, 42 percent more manganese, 9 percent more potassium, and 15 percent fewer nitrates (see www.foodisyourbestmedicine.com). Organically grown crops of spinach, lettuce, cabbage, and potatoes, for instance, showed even higher nutritional superiority. According to a USDA study, because of the mineral depletion of commercial crop soil, you would have to eat 72 servings of spinach today to get the same amount of minerals that you got in just one serving in 1948.

Not Only Fruits and Vegetables

The health reasons for going organic are numerous, and not just for produce. Animals raised organically are not given hormones, growth stimulants, or routine antibiotics. Since these drugs accumulate in the animal's tissue, when we eat non-organic meat, we are consuming them. Experts agree that, by putting substances such as antibiotics in animal feed, conventional farmers are stimulating the emergence of drug-resistant bacteria and contributing to a generation of children becoming antibiotic resistant. This resistance can have extreme repercussions in the face of a serious illness. The US Center for Disease Control has said that antibiotic resistance is one of the world's most pressing health problems. Already over 10,000 people in the United States die each year due to resistant strains of bacteria. Eating meat from an animal raised with antibiotics may put you at risk of contracting a drug-resistant bug directly from the meat; it may also make it harder for you to be treated for an illness that would easily have been cured in the past. The Union of Concerned Scientists as well as the AMA and the Institute for Agriculture and Trade Policy are now joining many other consumer groups rallying to support legislation introduced by Senator Edward Kennedy aimed at reducing the use of antibiotics on healthy livestock. Until such legislation is passed and implemented, I'd recommend that, if you're going to eat meat, choose organic.

Growth Hormones

Consumption of secondhand growth hormones and growth stimulants found in meat and dairy has been linked to premature development. Many studies have shown that school-age children are developing at a much earlier age than those of prior generations. Think back to what nine year olds looked like when you were in fourth grade, and compare that to how they look today.

Twice a month, genetically engineered recumbent Bovine Growth Hormone (rBGH) is injected into over three million dairy cows in the United States to stimulate their milk production. Although the FDA has concluded that this milk is safe for human consumption, recent studies challenge this conclusion.

When the FDA approved rBGH, it relied almost exclusively on an unpublished study by Monsanto, the world's largest producer of rBGH. In Canada, scientists working for the health protection branch of the government spotted the bias and reviewed the data, coming up with startlingly different conclusions. They found that consumption of the recumbent Bovine Growth Hormone led to cysts in the thyroid and higher levels of the hormone in the prostate. In addition, there is now evidence that rBGH might be a contributing factor in breast and prostate cancers in humans. In 2001, a US consumer group called the Center for Food Safety began legal action to have the hormone pulled off the market, claiming that the US Food and Drug Administration is ignoring evidence of potential health hazards from rBGH.

Furthermore, the extra milk production caused by rBGH makes cows more likely to develop udder infections called mastitis. One symptom of mastitis is large amounts of pus or blood in cow's milk. The main effect of higher pus levels is a higher infection rate, which, in turn, leads to increased antibiotic use in the cows. Milk on our grocery store shelves from rBGH-injected cows could contain residues of more than 80 different drugs, many of them used to treat sick animals.

Since our children are the first generation to act as guinea pigs, no one really knows what the long-term effects of ingesting these hormones will be, especially in combination with pesticide residues. What's a concerned parent to do? Look for milk labeled "BGH Free," or switch to soy or rice milk on your cereal.

Contributing to the Future of Our Planet

Many people who eat organic foods believe that the sustainable agricultural practices of organic farmers are the very key to our survival. Organic food is grown not only without the use of pesticides but also without petroleum- or sewage-based fertilizers, bioengineering, or ionizing radiation.

Bob Scrowcroft of the non-profit Organic Farming Research Foundation explains that our current agricultural system was implemented in the 1950s when farmers first discovered that chemical fertilizers could yield greater crops and synthetic pesticides could destroy more pests. However, as renewable agricultural practices became a distant memory, the insects that died off easily at first left behind some survivors, and within a few generations whole populations of insects became resistant. "Today we're applying three times as much chemicals as we were 40 years ago to kill the same pests," Scrowcroft says. And not just fertilizers are now destroying the soil: farmers use herbicides to kill weeds, fungicides to kill fungi, rodenticides to kill mice, and avicides to kill fruit-eating birds. These chemicals are showing up in our food supply and are killing off wildlife—not to mention endangering farm workers and destroying groundwater. When I lived in Iowa, known to have the most contaminated groundwater of any state because of farmers' dependence on chemical fertilizers and insecticides for soy and corn crops, not more than two or three months went by without another of my friends being diagnosed with cancer or other diseases directly related to toxic poisoning—and the population of the town was only 12,000.

Pesticides kill 67 million birds in the United States each year. The Mississippi River dumps enough synthetic fertilizer into the Gulf of Mexico to maintain a 60-mile-wide "dead zone" too overgrown with algae to support any aquatic life. Pesticide and fertilizer residues are left in the air for all creatures to breathe, and these residues can take years, decades, and sometimes even centuries to break down.

The word *organic* on a food product label stands for commitment to an agriculture that strives for a balance with nature. Farmers who use organic growing methods and people who buy organic foods are committed to long-term care of the land. Their mission is to ensure the sustainability of agriculture through care of the air, soil, and water. People who buy organic foods also want to maintain the health of people, plants, and animals. Whenever you have a choice, choose organic over conventional fruits, vegetables, and even meats. The cost might be higher, but your family's health and the future of our planet are worth it. And, truthfully, in our family we firmly believe that our outstanding health can largely be attributed not only to our vegetarian lifestyle but also to our organic choices.

Some Final Food for Thought
Genetically Modified Organisms (GMOs) in Our Food Supply

The genetic manipulation of food and its potentially devastating implications are a mounting controversy. Only a small percentage of the population is paying attention to this debate. Meanwhile, genetically modified foods are sneaking onto grocery store shelves. Approximately 60 percent of the soy and 38 percent of the corn planted in the United States has been genetically altered. In addition, most of the canola oil in the US market and many, if not most, commercially produced fruits and vegetables have now been genetically altered. Given the prevalence of soy and corn in processed foods, chances are you're already consuming a lot of genetically modified food without even knowing it, especially since the USFDA doesn't require stating GMO use on the label.

What is genetically modified food? Genetic engineering is a form of plant breeding radically different from anything that humans have ever practiced. In this process, genes from one species are synthetically inserted into a different species with which it would not naturally breed. By genetically modifying or engineering a certain plant, scientists hope to change its DNA. For example, scientists may take a cold-resistant gene from a jellyfish and insert it into a peach in an attempt to make the fruit heartier under colder growing conditions. Sound like something from a horror film?

Think about how hard it is to truly be a vegetarian these days. Eat a potato chip and you've probably broken your commitment to strict vegetarian practices. As for adherents of religions that eschew certain food categories, well, it's up to them to decide if they should eat soybeans that could contain genes from a pig.

Proponents of genetic engineering claim that it is the solution to world hunger. Their platform is that GMOs will feed the world, protect the environment by decreasing our dependence on certain agricultural chemicals, and help farmers to produce more with lower input costs. Most importantly, they insist that GMOs are not dangerous.

Opponents disagree. Many serious public health concerns have been raised in Europe and elsewhere. Scientists against GMOs are concerned about the possibility of new allergens being introduced in genetically modified foods. Take the frost-resistant peach as an example: if you are allergic to fish and eat a peach that contains a fish gene, you might have an allergic reaction and not have a clue what caused it.

In 1999, a major lawsuit against the FDA uncovered documents showing that its scientists concluded that genetically engineered foods do, in fact, pose unique safety hazards and recommended that each one be subjected to rigorous safety testing. These warnings by the FDA's best scientists are still being ignored. The worldwide alarm about the safety of genetically altered food, for both human health and the environment, has reached a monumental pitch for those who care to listen. In the European Union and particularly Great Britain, citizens have stated that they simply do not want these foods grown in their countries or put on their dinner tables. In response to huge consumer demand and grassroots consumer efforts, all major supermarket chains and food companies in Europe have removed genetically engineered foods from their shelves. In May 2002, the prestigious 115,000-member British Medical Association (equivalent to the AMA in the United States) issued a report that called for a nationwide moratorium on such foods and crops. Even Prince Charles has been a vocal opponent of GMOs.

As hard as this is to believe, there are no laws in the US requiring safety testing for GMO foods. The US regulatory agencies (USDA, FDA, EPA) have relied until now solely on tests done by the companies that make genetically engineered products to endorse their safety. These companies conduct only voluntary testing, and there are many questions that in-house testing doesn't ask.

I believe that taking genes from one species and putting them into another isn't "substantially equivalent" to anything else we've ever done on this planet. When the biotech industry develops corn genetically engineered with a bacterial toxin that acts as a insecticide, am I supposed to eat an ear of that corn and feel confident that it won't harm me? How can I, or anyone else, possibly know the long-term effects when we have been consuming these foods only for the past few years? If I become ill, how will my physician be able to connect cause and effect without my knowing what I've really been ingesting?

The consequences of consuming these novel products are completely unknown. The results may include harm to the immune system, triggering of autoimmune disease, and induction of allergic responses; further evolution of antibiotic resistance in pathogenic germs from the use of antibiotic resistance marker genes commonly used in most genetically modified products; and reduction of beneficial phytoestrogen levels.

One Swedish study suggests that the incidence of foodborne diseases in Sweden in 1994 was similar to that of the United States, which isn't surprising since the countries are comparable in their food hygiene. But since then the incidence of food-borne disease in the United States has undergone a tenfold increase. Notably, production of genetically engineered food has increased enormously in the United States since 1994, and, while viruses have been shown to cause only nine percent of the documented cases in Sweden, they have caused 80 percent of the cases in the United States. Thus, according to health authorities, we should be on the lookout for new viruses and bacteria that could evolve by the horizontal transfer and recombination of viral and bacterial genes in genetically engineered crops.

According to a report published at the end of 1999 by P.S. Mead and colleagues, food-borne diseases cause approximately 76 million illnesses, 325,000 hospitalizations, and 5,000 deaths in the United States each year. Known food-borne pathogens account for 14 million of the illnesses, 60,000 hospitalizations, and 1,800 deaths. In other words, unknown agents account for approximately 81 percent of food-borne illnesses and hospitalizations and 64 percent of deaths.

As for genetically engineered crops being the answer to world hunger, I think that Dr. Mae-Wan Ho, director of the Institute of Science in Society, London, England, states the facts far better than I could possibly restate them:

Open Letter to New Zealand Royal Commission on Genetic Engineering From:

Dr. Mae-Wan Ho
Director, Institute of Science in Society
PO Box 32097, London NW1 0XR

UK August 13, 2001

As one of the many scientists presenting evidence to the Royal Commission on Genetic Engineering, I had high hopes that New Zealand would assume moral and intellectual leadership in rejecting this dangerous technology bolstered by degenerate science, so obviously serving the corporate agenda instead of the public good. It is still not too late for New Zealand to take on this role. It has become increasingly evident that GM technology is inherently hazardous and unreliable both in agriculture and in medicine. The list of failures is growing apace. Let me mention a few recent examples that came to light since I presented evidence to the Commission. GM crops are inherently unstable, and this is fully borne out by numerous new scientific publications. Even the top success, Roundup Ready soya, is showing every sign of breakdown including reduced yield, non-germination, diseases and infestation by new pests. Molecular genetic characterization, the first ever done on any commercially grown GM crop so far, has confirmed that both the GM construct of Roundup Ready soya and the host genome have been scrambled (rearranged), and hundreds of base-pairs of unknown DNA has got in as well.

The "next generation" crops are even worse. I draw your attention especially to those developed with terminator technologies aimed at protecting corporate patents and preventing farmers from saving and replanting seeds. Many are currently field tested and commercially grown as "male sterile" crops. Not only are the constructs more complicated and hence more unstable and prone to horizontal gene transfer, the gene products used are cell poisons or recombinases, i.e., genome scramblers. Female-sterile and even male-sterile genes (yes!) are being spread via pollen. These dangerous genes will spread and wipe out other crops as well as wild plant species. It has become all too clear that GM agriculture cannot co-exist with other forms of agriculture. Bees are known to travel up to 10km or more in foraging for pollen. And there is no way to prevent the horizontal spread of GM constructs to unrelated species, which can occur in all environments, including the digestive and respiratory tracts of animals, as stated in evidence I have already presented. . . . A sweeping paradigm change is long overdue if we are to survive the destruction that reductionist science and technology have wrought on us and on our planet. We have all the means to deliver genuine health and food security to the world without using GM technology and going against the wishes of the vast majority of people. Only the political will is missing.

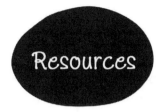

The International Vegetarian Union

www.ivu.org

In 1908, this non-profit organization replaced the Vegetarian Federal Union, established in 1889. Its goal is to bring together vegetarian societies from all parts of the world. The site features articles, recipes, famous vegetarians, vegetarian phrases in many languages, and international events. There are also discussion and news forums.

Veggilicious

www.veggilicious.com

Veggilicious.com is an informative and easy-to-use vegetarian and vegan restaurant directory currently focused on the Washington, DC, area. If you are looking for a good vegetarian meal in a friendly restaurant, this is the first place you should check. You want a restaurant that not only offers vegetarian meals but also treats vegetarians and vegans as valued customers. The site doesn't list any restaurant that isn't vegetarian friendly.

Vegging Out!

http://my.execpc.com/~veggie/index.html

Vegging Out! is dedicated to promoting plant-based food and nutrition, whether you are a vegan, vegetarian, or someone who simply wants to eat more foods from the earth. There's a great section just for kids.

North American Vegetarian Society

www.navs-online.org

This non-profit educational organization promotes the health, nutritional, environmental, and compassionate benefits of a meatless diet. It organizes the annual Vegetarian Summerfest.

Vegan Action

www.vegan.org

A non-profit educational organization based in Berkeley, California, Vegan Action has set up a site that caters to vegans. It's full of information, including the latest issue of *Vegan News*, a catalog of T-shirts, stickers, zines, and cookbooks, and information on joining the latest vegan campaign.

Animal Concerns

www.animalconcerns.org

The Animal Concerns Community is a project of the EnviroLink Network, a non-profit organization that has been providing access to thousands of on-line environmental and animal rights/welfare resources since 1991. This community serves as a clearinghouse for information on the Internet related to animal rights and welfare.

Gourmet Vegetarians

www.gourmet-vegetarian.com

This not-for-profit web site provides vegetarian links and resources for vegans, vegetarians, and those considering a vegetarian lifestyle. The extensive vegetarian cooking glossary of terms is a very helpful tool for learning all about vegetarianism and gourmet cooking. A glossary of herbs is on its way too.

Teen Vegetarian

www.geocities.com/HotSprings/2657

Teen Vegetarian is a web page on all aspects of the vegetarian movement, written entirely by and for vegetarian teens. You can find everything from information on vegetarian bands to all the reasons that vegetarians detest McDonald's.

Famous Veggies

www.famousveggie.com

The purpose of the famous vegetarians site is to demonstrate how widespread vegetarianism is becoming around the world. The great number of vegetarians who are famous show how many people are becoming educated and realizing that it is the sensible way to live. The site is meant to be informative and educational. Plus it's fun to see all the people whom you might not have known were or are vegetarian.

Vegetarian Tips

www.vegetarian-tips.com/About.asp

Filled with vegetarian tips!

Vegetarian Kitchen

www.vegkitchen.com

Step into the kitchen of Nava Atlas, author and illustrator of many books on vegetarian cooking. The best known are *Vegetariana, Vegetarian Soups for all Seasons, Vegetarian Express,* and *Vegetarian Celebrations.* Her articles on healthy cooking with natural foods have appeared in *Vegetarian Times, Veggie Life, Great Life,* and other magazines and newspapers.

Vegetarian Store

www.vegetarianstore.com

Vegetarianstore.com offers delicious food choices for people interested in a healthier, meatless, and low-cholesterol but great-tasting diet. Meat lovers and vegetarians alike will enjoy these vegetarian soy meats and milk alternatives. Vegetarianstore. com offers top-quality products.

Veggie Dates

www.veggiedate.org

Veggie Dates is the premier vegetarian and vegan singles dating service. Search and place personal ads, find pen pals, and enjoy ongoing associations with hundreds of vegetarian, vegan, macrobiotic, raw food, animal protection, and environmental organizations.

Vegetarian Source

www.vegsource.com

This site offers a lot of information and links regarding all facets of vegetarianism. It is hosted by VegSource and is an Internet partner with the International Vegetarian Union.

Jewish Vegan Lifestyle

http://jewishvegan.com

The purpose of jewishvegan.com is to promote the practice of a vegan lifestyle within the Torah laws, both written and oral.

Vegan Outreach

www.veganoutreach.org

This organization works to end animal exploitation by promoting a vegan lifestyle. Its main activity is distributing a booklet called *Why Vegan?* that goes beyond the simple definition of veganism by showing individuals how to better the world through their daily choices. The site also provides essays, newsletters, resources, and links.

Vegan Society

www.vegansociety.com

This charitable organization is located in the United Kingdom and promotes "ways of living which avoid the use of animal products — for the benefit of people, animals and the environment." It is a great source for travel tips in England, Scotland, Wales, and Ireland. You can also find links to other vegan sites, products, books, information sheets, and news.

The Vegetarian Society UK

www.vegsoc.org

The Vegetarian Society of the United Kingdom is celebrating its 150th year. There is information on new vegetarian recipes, health and nutrition, a local directory, animal rights, books, and a lot more. It's a comprehensive site overall, with a lot of information for vegetarians young and old, new and experienced.

The Vegetarian Youth Network

www.geocities.com/RainForest/Vines/4482

The Vegetarian Youth Network is a grassroots organization run entirely for and by teenagers who support vegetarian living. The group sponsors a help line for information, products, and directories of information.

Vegan Street

www.veganstreet.com

The site includes information and news.

For New Vegetarians

www.newveg.av.org

This site is of specific interest to entry-level vegetarians. This virtual compendium of vegetarian information and sources allows you to look up "How to Be a Vegetarian in 10 Easy Steps," to cope with vegan dating dilemmas, and to scan the lyrics to "Meat Is Murder" by Morrissey.

The Vegetarian Pages
www.veg.org
This site intends to "be a definitive guide to what is available on the Internet for vegetarians, vegans, and others." Many links to vegetarian resources are found here.

The Vegetarian Resource Group
www.vrg.org
This is an extensive site with information on vegetarianism in a nutshell—the basic facts and how to become vegetarian. There are also lists of vegetarian literature and teaching materials, recipes, and food replacements. Check out the vegetarian search engine and feedback page for comments. Other topics include feeding vegan kids, a guide to non-leather goods, a lesson plan for teachers, vegetarian-friendly investing, and vegetarians on-line—links to finding vegetarian stuff on AOL, CompuServe, MSN, and other service providers.

Veggie Heaven
www.veggieheaven.com
This site is a great source of vegetarian information on the web. You can find over 230 of the tastiest vegetarian and vegan recipes, a UK vegetarian restaurant guide, facts and nutritional information, and lots more.

VegWeb

www.vegweb.com

This is an on-line guide to vegetarianism, including a number of bulletin boards on topics from animal rights to parenting. There are also book reviews and information on composting and meal planning.

Daysworth

www.daysworth.com

Daysworth.com is the world's first and most comprehensive nutritional search engine. Visitors can easily calculate the nutritional value of a specific food, a meal, or even a whole day's menu. Find out whether or not you are getting the proper day's worth of vitamins, minerals, protein, and other important nutrients. Daysworth not only gives a complete nutritional breakdown of the essential nutrients in foods but also provides links to the web sites of food manufacturers listed.

FATFREE: The Low Fat Vegetarian Recipe Archive

www.fatfree.com

This site provides numerous low-fat vegetarian recipes. You can search the archive, check out newly submitted recipes, and access the USDA nutrient database. It also offers some interaction by allowing users to submit recipes for posting.

Living Foods

www.living-foods.com

This site serves to educate people about the power of living and raw foods. It provides background information, recipes, articles, message boards, chatrooms, resources, a marketplace, and a search engine.

Moosewood Restaurant

www.moosewoodrestaurant.com

The Moosewood Restaurant in Ithaca, New York, is one of the oldest vegetarian restaurants in the United States. Its site has free vegetarian recipes, on-line ordering for its cookbooks, and information about its consulting work and cooking lessons.

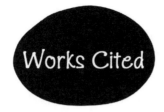

Works Cited

Allen, Lindsay H., et al. "Protein-Induced Hypercalciuria: A Longer Term Study." *American Journal of Clinical Nutrition* 32 (1979): 741–49.

American Cancer Society. "Cancer Facts and Figures." www.cancer.org/docroot/STT/stt_0.asp

August, Melissa, et al. "Should We All Be Vegetarians?" *Time* 15 July 2002: 48–56.

Barzel, U. "The Effects of Excessive Acid Feeding on Bone." *Calc Tiss Res* 4 (1969): 94.

Bezkorovainy, A., and D.M. Czajka-Narins. *Biochemistry of Nonheme Iron*. New York: Plenum, 1980.

Brockis, J. "The Effects of Vegetable and Animal Protein Diets on Calcium, Urate, and Oxalate Excretion." *Br J Urology* 54 (1982): 590.

Campbell, T. Colin. "Muscling Out the Meat Myth." www.vsdc.org/meatmyth.html

Claude-Chang, J., et al. "Mortality Pattern of German Vegetarians after 11 Years of Follow-Up." *Epidemiology* 3.5 (1992): 395–401.

Croft, J.B., et al. "Transitions of Cardiovascular Risk from Adolescence to Young Adulthood: The Bogalusa Heart Study. I. Effects of Alterations in Lifestyle." *Journal of Chronic Diseases* 39 (1986): 81–90.

Doll, R. "Symposium on Diet and Cancer." *Proceedings of the Nutrition Society* 49 (1990): 119–31.
www.vegetarian-diet.info/cancer-vegetarian-health.htm

EarthSave spring 1997.

Emerson, Tony. "Where's the Beef?" *Newsweek* 26 Feb. 2001: 12–17.

Flores, Alfredo. "Breakfast Is Key to Achieving Maximum Nutrition." USDA Agricultural Research Service Online Article. 21 June 2002.
www.ars.usda.gov/is/pr/2002/020621.htm

The Food and Nutrition Information Center (FNIC).
www.nal.usda.gov/fnic/

Ho, Mae-Wan. "Cloning and ES Cells Both Biting the Dust." *ISIS Report* 11 July 2001.
www.gefree.org.nz/maewhoopltr.htm

Ho, Mae-Wan, and Joe Cummins. "Terminate the Terminators." *ISIS Report* 23 July 2001.
www.gefree.org.nz/maewhoopltr.htm

— ."Xeno-Transplantation: How Bad Science and Big Business Put the World at Risk from Viral Pandemics." *ISIS Sustain-able Science*, Audit 2, Aug. 2000.
www.gefree.org.nz/maewhoopltr.htm

Japenga, Ann. "Mending the Female Heart." *Health* Mar. 1996: 8–72.

Journal of the American Dietetic Association 97.11 (1997): 1317.

Journal of the National Cancer Institute 84 (1992): 1461.

Kolata, Gina. "Major Study Links Animal Fats to Cancer of Colon." *New York Times* 13 Dec. 1990.

Kradjian, Robert. *Save Yourself from Breast Cancer.* New York: Berkley, 1994.

Krizmanic, Judy. "Riding the Calcium Roller Coaster." *Vegetarian Times* July 1995: 63.

— . *A Teen's Guide to Going Vegetarian.* New York: Penguin, 1994.

Lappe, Frances Moore. *Diet for a Small Planet.* Rev. ed. New York: Ballantine, 1982.

Liebman, Bonnie. "Calcium: After the Craze." *Nutrition Action Health Letter* June 1994: 8.

— . "Pesticides and Breast Cancer." *Nutrition Action Health Letter* Mar. 1999.

Mead, P.S., et al. "Food-Related Illness and Death in the United States." *Emerging Infectious Diseases* 5 (1999): 607–25.

Messina, M., and V. Messina. *The Dietitian's Guide to Vegetarian Diets: Issues and Applications.* Gaithersburg, MD: Gage, 1996.

Messina, V.L., and K.I. Burke. "Position of the American Dietetic Association: Vegetarian Diets." *Journal of the American Dietetic Association* (1997): 1317–21.

The National Academy of Science's Food and Nutrition Board. www4.nas.edu/IOM/IOMHome.nsf/Pages/Food+and+Nutrition+Board

Northrup, Christiane. *Women's Bodies, Women's Wisdom*. New York: Bantam, 1994.

Ornish, Dean. *Dr. Dean Ornish's Program for Reversing Heart Disease*. New York: Ballantine, 1990.

Parker, F.C., et al. "The Association between Cardiovascular Response Tasks and Future Blood Pressure Levels in Children: Bogalusa Heart Study." *American Heart Journal* 113 (1987): 1174–79.

Paul, Jacquie. "Study Backs Adventist Lifestyle: A Loma Linda University Researcher Cites an Avoidance of Meat and Alcohol for Longer Life Spans." *Press Enterprise, Riverside and San Bernardino Counties*, 10 July 2001.
http://tofu. org/pipermail/tofu/2001–July/000033.html

Reeser, Cyndi. Excerpt from "Issues in Vegetarian Dietetics." *Animal Writes Online Newsletter* 5 Nov. 2000.
www.geocities.com/RainForest/1395/aro001105.html

Robbins, John. *Diet for a New America*. Walpole, NH: Stillpoint, 1987.

Robertson, W. "The Effect of High Protein Intake on the Risk of Calcium Stone Formation in the Urinary Tract." *Clinical Science* 57 (1979): 285.

Robinson, Simon. "Grains of Hope." *Time* 31 July 2000: 38–46.

Vegetarian Nutrition.
www.vegetariannutrition. net/ articles.htm

Vegetarian Resource Group.
www.vrg.org

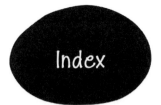

Index